University of Brighton

Falmer Library
Falmer
Brighton BN1 9PH
Telephone 01273 643570

Online renewal http://library.brighton.ac.uk

ealthcare:

)r John Fulton

Please return or renew on or before the last date stamped
A fine may be charged if items are returned late

IS_02.01.14.ISR.

Full the full range of M&K Publishing books please visit our website:

www.mkupdate.co.uk

Studying Postgraduate Healthcare

A pre-reader

Edited by Dr Catherine Hayes and Dr John Fulton

Studying Postgraduate Healthcare: A pre reader

Catherine Hayes
John Fulton
(editors)

ISBN: 9781905539-99-4

First published 2015

British Library Cataloguing in Publication Data

A catalogue record for this book is available from the British Library

Notice

Clinical practice and medical knowledge constantly evolve. Standard safety precautions must be followed, but, as knowledge is broadened by research, changes in practice, treatment and drug therapy may become necessary or appropriate. Readers must check the most current product information provided by the manufacturer of each drug to be administered and verify the dosages and correct administration, as well as contraindications. It is the responsibility of the practitioner, utilising the experience and knowledge of the patient, to determine dosages and the best treatment for each individual patient. Any brands mentioned in this book are as examples only and are not endorsed by the publisher. Neither the publisher nor the authors assume any liability for any injury and/or damage to persons or property arising from this publication.

Disclaimer

M&K Publishing cannot accept responsibility for the contents of any linked website or online resource. The existence of a link does not imply any endorsement or recommendation of the organisation or the information or views which may be expressed in any linked website or online resource. We cannot guarantee that these links will operate consistently and we have no control over the availability of linked pages.

To contact M&K Publishing write to:
M&K Update Ltd · The Old Bakery · St. John's Street
Keswick · Cumbria CA12 5AS
Tel: 01768 773030 · Fax: 01768 781099
publishing@mkupdate.co.uk
www.mkupdate.co.uk

Designed and typeset by Mary Blood
Printed by McKanes Printers, Keswick

Contents

About the contributors

Sonia Bussey

Sonia was appointed as Lecturer in Medical Education at the University of Newcastle in 2012. She is a Podiatrist by profession, and worked in the NHS in Oxfordshire and Gateshead before becoming an academic at the Durham School of Podiatric Medicine. Her current role is primarily focused on developing improved relationships and coherence between practice teachers for the MBBS programme and Newcastle University in the capacity of a clinical co-ordinator.

Dr John Fulton

Dr John Fulton is Principal Lecturer in Health in the Department of Pharmacy, Health and Well-being at the University of Sunderland. He is interested in the application of theoretical issues from social science to health and sport and in the interaction of formal learning with non-formal and informal learning. John teaches on a variety of programmes in the Faculty of Applied Sciences and is a member of the core team for the University's professional doctorate scheme, where he leads on the research methods module. He is interested in learning in the workplace and is module leader for Evidence-Based Healthcare and Teaching and Assessing in Clinical Practice. He also teaches on modules relating sociological theory to health and sport.

Dr Catherine Hayes

Catherine is a Principal Lecturer within the Department of Pharmacy, Health and Well-being in the Faculty of Applied Sciences at the University of Sunderland. Her research and scholarly activity is embedded within both the strategic institutional focus of the Centre for Pedagogy and the Faculty of Applied Sciences Research Beacon. She has published widely within the context of allied healthcare curricula and on the need for professional capacity building within and between professional disciplines. She has also contributed to interprofessional knowledge sharing in advancing clinical practice for healthcare practitioners. Catherine is a UK Regional Adviser in Podiatric Medicine for the Royal College of Physicians and Surgeons in Glasgow.

Shelagh Keogh

Shelagh has been a member of academic staff at Northumbria University since 2000, having studied Information Technology at the University of Sunderland. Her research interests include professionalism in practice, teaching and learning in technology and project management (both generally and with sociology). Shelagh describes teaching and contact with students as the most enjoyable part of her job. She currently teaches Project Management, Professionalism, Systems Analysis, Effective Systems Development and Strategic Management.

Dr Judith Kuit

Judith was a researcher in Renal Physiology at Newcastle's Medical School. She moved to Sunderland to lecture, becoming the Faculty Teaching and Learning Co-ordinator and the University's Head of Academic Development. She has a particular interest in distance and e-learning and has become a Visiting Professor of E-learning in Bahrain. Judith is one of the core team supporting Sunderland's professional doctorate programme and is currently leading curriculum developments for the University in healthcare science, alongside clinical colleagues both locally and nationally. Judith's current research interests are pedagogical. She is interested in student-centred learning, particularly supporting off-campus learners who may be in the workplace or geographically separated.

Shelagh Keogh

Shelagh has been a member of academic staff at Northumbria University since 2000, having studied Information Technology at the University of Sunderland. Her research interests include professionalism in practice, teaching and learning in technology and project management (both generally and with sociology). Shelagh describes teaching and contact with students as the most enjoyable part of her job. She currently teaches Project Management, Professionalism, Systems Analysis, Effective Systems Development and Strategic Management.

Professor Peter Smith

Professor Peter Smith is Emeritus Professor of Computing at the University of Sunderland. He joined the University as an undergraduate student in 1975 and received his Doctorate in 1981. Since then he has held several teaching, research and management positions at the University, including Dean, and Chair of the University Research Degrees Committee. He has published over 250 papers, and supervised and examined over 100 doctoral candidates at universities in the UK, Europe and Hong Kong. Peter is a Fellow of the British Computer Society and the Higher Education Academy. He has published extensively on a range of subjects including computing, management and doctoral studies, particularly in relation to professional doctorates.

Preface

As academics with long experience of dealing with new postgraduate healthcare students, we felt there was a need to provide a readable resource for people contemplating a postgraduate educational pathway in healthcare. In this book we have deliberately adopted an accessible, non-academic style, although the content is evidence based. We hope it will provide a much-needed overview of the practical considerations that should be taken into account when embarking on any postgraduate healthcare course.

We have designed the book to be read as a quick overview of the whole process so that it is essentially an 'easy read' for those developing their thinking about study in general, and studying at master's and doctoral-level specifically. The chapters can also be read independently and readers can dip into them, as they wish.

Above all, we hope this book will show that educational institutions care about their students in a holistic sense, as human beings. This is significant when we consider the huge impact that undertaking an educational journey in postgraduate healthcare can have on everyday life, and the accompanying need to manage the changes it brings. We believe that long-term education should be seen as an integral part of life, and not something that exists separately from the individual's normal existence.

During our careers as educationalists, it has been our privilege to work with students from all over the world. We would like to extend our thanks to them all for the insights and perspectives they have given us, which we now offer in this short book.

Dr Catherine Hayes and Dr John Fulton

1

Managing expectations in postgraduate education

Professor Peter Smith

This book is aimed at students who intend to follow a postgraduate qualification in health studies. This first chapter will survey the postgraduate education landscape, discuss what is meant by postgraduate standards, and look at what you might expect, should you choose to become a postgraduate student. In doing so, I hope to help you decide if a postgraduate programme is for you. If you decide that it is, you can begin to consider which type of programme is best suited to your needs.

After you have finished reading this chapter you should have a better understanding of the nature of postgraduate study, understand the difference between a master's degree and a doctorate, and be able to weigh up and consider the different reasons for studying as a postgraduate. You should also understand what you might expect from a postgraduate programme, and be in a position to decide whether or not postgraduate study is for you.

What is postgraduate education?

The term 'postgraduate' implies that you already have an initial or bachelor's degree (or its equivalent), and that you have chosen to undertake further study at a more advanced level. This suggests that you are, to some extent, hooked on learning and are a 'lifelong learner'. In general, there are two levels of postgraduate qualification; these are master's degrees such as Master of Arts (MA), Master of Science (MSc) and Master of Education (MEd); and doctorates, normally a PhD (Doctor of Philosophy) or a Professional Doctorate (DProf, DBA, EdD).

There are many different types of master's degrees and no nationally agreed definitions (QAA 2010). Master's degrees are often categorised as 'taught' or 'research'. A taught degree will include a lecture-based component in which the student learns some new, advanced, material. This will normally be followed by a substantial research project. A taught master's will normally take one year of full-time study, or two years of part-time study. A research master's will usually consist of a substantial (usually one to two years full-time) supervised research project and the production of a dissertation, or thesis, which presents and discusses the results of the research project.

A doctorate is a research degree, and is the highest level of academic qualification. Traditionally the standard doctoral qualification has been the PhD (Doctor of Philosophy). However, in recent years a new form of practitioner-based doctorate has emerged (Fulton *et al.* 2013), known as the professional doctorate (D Prof). The professional doctorate allows experienced practitioners to develop a research project within their own professional practice, and is a more work-based qualification. It thus offers several advantages for health professionals (Fulton *et al.* 2012). As with the PhD, it is a research degree and meets the same high academic standards.

In order to study for a doctorate, you will need to have a 'good' first degree (usually defined as a first-class or upper second-class honours degree) and, in some cases, a master's degree. In order to study for a professional doctorate, you will also normally be required to have substantial professional experience. There are also subject-based professional doctorate qualifications such as EdD (education), DBA (business) and EngD (Engineering).

There is a growing expectation that university research should result in benefits or 'impact' for business, health and society. The UK Research Evaluation Framework (REF 2014) defines impact as 'an effect on, change or benefit to the economy, society, culture, public policy or services, health, the environment or quality of life, beyond academia'. Form this point of view, the benefits of applied research have been recognised for many years (Smith & Elliott 1995). It is therefore quite likely that you will be able to develop a research project that links with your workplace or career aspirations, as more and more universities are looking for practical projects that result in concrete practitioner outcomes.

Taught programmes will be led by tutors, and you will be expected to attend regular lectures and seminars. There will also be a significant emphasis on independent learning; more so than in your first degree. Taught programmes are usually divided into modules and you will be assessed by means of a mixture of examinations, coursework and a large project or dissertation. Research degrees mainly rely on independent study, with support from an academic supervisor who you will meet at intervals to discuss progress on your research project.

Many universities are now offering students the opportunity to follow postgraduate programmes through distance learning. As the name suggests, you register to follow a degree with a university as an external student, many miles away from home, and often in another country. Distance learning can take many forms, and usually involves studying at home using online or printed materials, email and Skype. You may also be expected to visit a local study centre to meet tutors who will support you in your studies. Most distance learning programmes allow you to study on a part-time basis, which may enable you to continue working at the same time.

Distance learning programmes are usually flexible and allow you to study at your own pace, and from home (Becker 2004). However, this does require a great deal of self-discipline and dedication. You will not have the same level of face-to-face contact with tutors or the support of a peer group of fellow students. Many different distance-learning programmes are now being offered in several aspects of health studies. For example, Sowan and Jenkins (2013) describe the design of a distance learning programme for nurses, while Gemmell *et al.* (2011) present their experience of teaching biostatistics in an online Master of Public Health programme.

It is often assumed that postgraduate students are well versed in study, and the transition from undergraduate study to master's will be straightforward. However, Tobbell *et al.* (2013) question this and argue that the postgraduate experience has been largely ignored. Their findings suggest that postgraduate students lead complex lives and require specific and targeted support in their studies. This book aims to provide a resource that will help you choose, and prepare for, your postgraduate study programme.

Postgraduate standards (master's degrees and the doctorate)

The UK Quality Assurance Agency (QAA) framework for higher education qualifications in England, Wales and Northern Ireland (QAA 2008) describes the standard for a master's degree as:

- *A systematic understanding of knowledge, and a critical awareness of current problems and/or new insights, much of which is at, or informed by, the forefront of their academic discipline, field of study or area of professional practice*
- *A comprehensive understanding of techniques applicable to their own research or advanced scholarship*
- *Originality in the application of knowledge, together with a practical understanding of how established techniques of research and enquiry are used to create and interpret knowledge in the discipline*
- *Conceptual understanding that enables the student: to evaluate critically current research and advanced scholarship in the discipline, and to evaluate methodologies and develop critiques of them and, where appropriate, to propose new hypotheses.*

As the above suggests, studying for a master's degree involves learning about the latest work in your subject. It also usually involves a substantial research project, or dissertation, and the use of research methods to investigate an issue, or solve a problem, within your field of study. You will be expected to read a lot of recent and relevant material, to produce written work in the form of essays and a substantial project dissertation, and you may also have to sit some examinations. You will also be required to demonstrate the ability to write, and think, in a critical manner.

In a similar manner, the QAA (2008) describes the standard for a doctorate as:

- *The creation and interpretation of new knowledge, through original research or other advanced scholarship, of a quality to satisfy peer review, extend the forefront of the discipline, and merit publication*
- *A systematic acquisition and understanding of a substantial body of knowledge which is at the forefront of an academic discipline or area of professional practice*
- *The general ability to conceptualise, design and implement a project for the generation of new knowledge, applications or understanding at the forefront of the discipline, and to adjust the project design in the light of unforeseen problems*
- *A detailed understanding of applicable techniques for research and advanced academic enquiry.*

A master's degree normally takes one to two years of full-time study, while a doctorate normally takes at least three years. A doctorate always comprises a very substantial research project, while a master's often includes a taught component. The major difference between the master's degree and the doctorate is the concept of the 'contribution to knowledge', which is referred to as 'the creation and interpretation of new knowledge' in the QAA definition above. Taken literally, 'contribution to knowledge' means that the research project has resulted in something new, some findings that weren't known before your study, and some new knowledge that extends the subject discipline. This sounds quite daunting, but in practice isn't as grand as it sounds (Mullins & Kiley 2002). The other major difference is that the award of a doctorate enables the candidate to use the prefix 'Dr' before their name, signifying that they have reached the highest possible academic standard.

Choosing a study programme

There are certainly plenty of study programmes to choose from. The website **www.findamasters.com** lists 1,281 master's programmes in health sciences in the UK. No matter what your subject or professional interest, there is certain to be a programme available for you in a university somewhere. A quick search of a database of master's programmes reveals titles as diverse as MSc in Nursing and Midwifery, MSc Public Health Research, MSc Global Health and Management, MSc Physiotherapy, MSc in Biomedical Sciences, MSc in Clinical Health Management and MSc in Health Psychology. And there are lots more.

One way of finding out about the many different courses on offer is to attend a postgraduate study fair. These fairs are held regularly in major cities around the world. Whatever your reason for study (whether it is to improve your career prospects, because you wish to specialise in a particular field or simply because you enjoy studying), you will have many questions that you want answered. Attending a fair will enable you to talk to representatives from different universities and colleges, and to collect information about the many programmes available.

You can also seek advice from:

Lecturers: if you are a student at the moment you can talk to your tutors

Careers advisers: they will be aware of career prospects in your field, what you need to study, and will be able to discuss particular programmes impartially and perhaps suggest other options

Friends: if they have already gone on to postgraduate study, they will be able to tell you about their own experiences.

Motivation

Studying for a postgraduate degree can be a lengthy journey. You will be committing yourself to studying for one, two or more years, so you must be really sure that you want to do it. Everyone has their own reasons for opting to undertake further study. These may include:

Subject reasons: A postgraduate programme can help you to explore your personal interests. Many taught programmes allow you to select the modules you are most interested in, and you can pursue a particular interest in great depth during your project.

Career reasons: Gaining a postgraduate qualification may not have an immediate impact but, in the long term, it may well help you gain promotion and increase your earning potential. It may also enable you to gain new knowledge and skills so that you can change your career path. More than a quarter of graduates surveyed felt 'their future employment prospects were better as a result of their qualifications', according to a 2011 report by the Higher Education Statistics Agency (HESA) (Prospects website 2013).

Professional reasons: Some professions require a postgraduate qualification, and some programmes are combined with a professional qualification. For example, my daughter is currently studying a Master's in Social Work which, when completed, will qualify her to become a social worker. Her particular programme is two years full time and includes two substantial work placements.

Personal satisfaction: Maybe you are simply a true lifelong learner, who gains satisfaction from studying, learning new things and achieving qualifications.

Whatever your own motivations and goals, you need to be sure that you have a solid set of reasons for doing postgraduate study before you make any firm commitment to it. You have to be totally committed to the programme and to achieving the qualification. You must be feeling very positive indeed about studying, so much so that you get a buzz every time you return to your studies. Being half-hearted just isn't good enough and won't get you through those long, hard days when things aren't going quite as you would like. You must really want to do this and it has to be something that you are hungry for! If you are intending to study in order to improve your career prospects, choose your programme carefully, and check the entry requirements and career path that it prepares you for.

I asked some of my own students why they chose to undertake further study. The results of this small survey are shown in Figure 1.1 (below). You can see that the most popular response was: 'For a sense of personal achievement'. The next most popular choice was 'For subject/professional interest'.

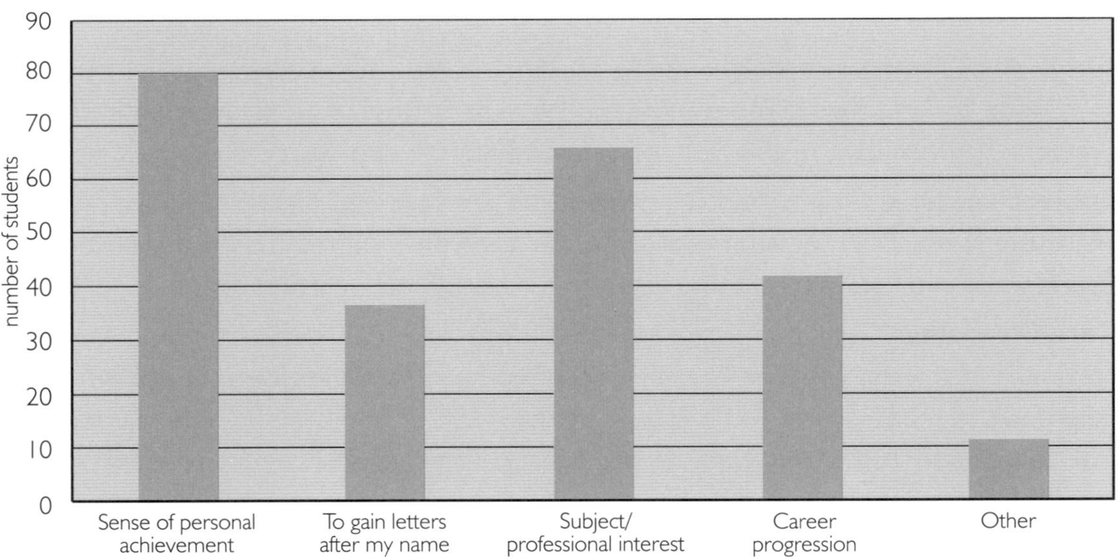

Figure 1.1: Reasons for undertaking postgraduate study

Here is a selection of comments from some of the students about their experiences:

- *'What I did not realise was the personal journey I would undergo and how it would affect the way I operate today.'*
- *'The first thing you must appreciate is the time and dedication necessary. There are no short cuts, there is no hiding place but the satisfaction of achieving your goal is immense. You will experience great comfort and satisfaction that you have completed a major piece of work, of which research is a fundamental part.'*
- *'This has been a difficult journey; juxtaposing a full-time senior management career and personal family commitments whilst at the same time trying to mesh in a demanding project. My knowledge and understanding of the subject, however, would not have been anywhere near as developed had I not embarked on this programme of study. I feel a real sense of achievement in being able to juggle so many demands and at the same time still managing to deliver the required outcomes to timescale.'*
- *'When I embarked on the programme, I had no clear expectations other than I wanted to see if I could achieve at this level of academic work. I can honestly say that if my work resulted in a fail that, whilst I would naturally be disappointed, I could walk away knowing that I have personally developed in a way that I never anticipated.'*
- *'Undertaking further study is not for the faint-hearted. You need to be very motivated, with big doses of perseverance, dedication and commitment and the ability to be absolutely determined to see it through to the end; the personal satisfaction when you are officially awarded your degree will make it one of the proudest days of your life.'*

Expectations

Much work has been done around the world to investigate how best to support students and thus increase student satisfaction. This includes the development of student charters or student contracts. These are formal agreements that set out exactly what students can expect from their university, and what the university expects of students.

Gaffney-Rhys & Jones (2010) considered the appropriateness of using student contracts. They found that such contracts were welcomed by students, and concluded that they could improve the service students receive, help students feel that they are valued members of an academic community, and increase student satisfaction. With the growing costs of attending university, many universities have considered the concept of 'students as customers' – as in a study carried out in Australia (Pitman 2000). Howell & Buck (2012) obtained feedback from 1,725 students and 214 lecturers at five institutions. Their study revealed that the four most important factors that affected adult students' satisfaction were:

relevance of subject-matter, staff competence, lecture management and student workload. Jancey & Burns (2013) undertook a case study of 51 taught postgraduate students on health programmes. Their study found that the students rated a number of factors as important to their studies. These included: the reputation of the university, the skills of the lecturers, access to online resources, and accessibility of staff.

The UK White Paper 'Higher Education: Students at the Heart of the System', which was presented to Parliament in June 2011, gives a commitment to: 'a renewed focus on high-quality teaching in universities … we will deliver a new focus on student charters, student feedback and graduate outcomes' (Thompson & Bekhradnia 2011). Universities actively seek out the views of their students. My own university has a university-wide project called 'Student Voice'. This is an inclusive commitment, which is communicated to all students through a variety of means. For instance, the university website includes the following wording:

> *We care about what our students think, so we have an on-going feedback system called 'Student Voice'. 'Student Voice' is how you can tell us what you think about specific issues – such as your course, the library service or the sports club – as well as how you feel about general issues relating to what life is like as a student. We collect your feedback in a variety of ways. Once we've collected everyone's feedback, we use it to try to improve your experience of university life. To see what changes we've made as a result of your feedback, look out for the 'Student Voice' notices on campus. You can also see summaries of all the changes we've made over the last year on the page 'You said it, We did it'.*

'Student Voice' is used to involve postgraduate students in all aspects of our programmes, including membership of our programme boards and participation in student surveys.

The UK Higher Education Academy runs national surveys of postgraduate students. For instance, PTES (Postgraduate Taught Experience Survey) is a national survey of postgraduate students in the UK, and allows institutions to collect feedback on the experiences of their taught postgraduate students. Likewise, the Postgraduate Research Experience Survey (PRES) collects data on the experience of postgraduate research students. The results of these surveys are discussed at our committees, and appropriate action taken in response. For example, in 2009 PRES told us (HEA 2013) that research students would welcome more seminars at university and faculty level, more social activities for students, and more flexible approaches to our training programmes. These issues were discussed in an open meeting with students, and together we devised an action plan. The actions were taken forward and communicated to the entire student body via our website, staff–student liaison meetings and our research student representatives.

Universities are seeking to engage with students and provide them with programmes to suit their needs. You should therefore make the most of these opportunities by working with the university of your choice, and taking part in any activities that enable you to exert your influence.

Information and Guidance (IAG)

Every university provides a lot of detail about their courses, and other aspects of university life, through their website. This will include full course details, details of the teaching, learning and assessment approaches, information on the social and sports provision, and details of accommodation and other student support services. This type of information is often referred to as 'Information and Guidance' or IAG.

The UK 1994 Group have produced a useful document called *Managing Students' Expectations of University* (Dunbar-Morris 2010). This includes several case studies looking at the different ways in which universities provide IAG. The 1994 Group has been established to 'promote excellence in university research and teaching, and represents 19 of the UK's leading research-intensive, student focused universities.'

They categorise IAG under the following four headings:

Capacity-building initiatives: These cover the development of prospective students' skills such as study skills. They provide opportunities to gain familiarity with the university environment before fully committing to a course. This might include doing some taster courses, perhaps online, which prepare you for university life.

The academic experience: This is about explaining the learning and teaching approaches on the course you are considering; the methods of assessment (including the balance of examination and coursework), and how the curriculum is organised (for instance, the balance between lecture and tutorials). All this information will be useful when you are choosing a programme.

Social experience: This covers the accommodation provided by the university or by private landlords, the students' union facilities, social and sports facilities, student clubs, and so on.

Professional services: These services include support for international students and careers guidance.

Whichever university or course you are considering, they will almost certainly offer plenty of IAG. Start by going to their website and do some research on the areas mentioned above. This may lead to further questions, which can be answered by emailing or telephoning the university. There are many texts, such as this one and Wilkinson (2005) and Wisker (2007), which you will find useful when you are looking for a programme to study.

Accreditation of Prior Learning (APL)

Accreditation of Prior Learning (or APL) is the process by which you can obtain credit towards a qualification by using something that you have learnt in the past. Many universities operate this process, which enables you to use credits that you have previously earned for your studies, or in some cases from previous work experience or training. This could mean that you will be exempted from certain modules or other parts of the study programme. To gain APL, you will be required to prove that you have undertaken the prior learning and that it is up to date and relevant to your new programme of study. The learning may be from a previous course, which was assessed and for which you have already gained a qualification. Or it may have been gained from practical experience while you were doing a job.

If you believe that some of your previous learning might count towards the programme that you are considering applying to, you will need to contact the university and enquire as to whether they operate an APL system. If they do, and they are able to consider your request, you will need to provide evidence showing that you have similar knowledge and skills to those covered in the part of the programme from which you are seeking exemption. There are limits to how much APL can be gained towards a programme, and the previous work you are using will need to be at the correct level. The university to which you are applying will be able to help you with this.

Choosing your programme

You need to consider all the aspects discussed above when choosing your postgraduate programme. Figure 1.2 provides a useful checklist. Hesketh & Knight (1999) encourage you to contact academic staff and to speak to other students so that you can discover something of the 'lived experience' of the programme that you are considering.

Conclusion

This chapter has introduced the concept of postgraduate study, and given you an idea of the different types of degree that are available. This should enable you to start to decide whether or not further study is for you. The following chapters will examine certain aspects of postgraduate study in greater detail, helping you to make an informed decision as to which way forward is best for you. Good luck with your studies, which I hope will prove to be challenging, rewarding and enjoyable.

Questions	
Which subject area do you wish to study?	
Which type of programme do you require (taught or research)?	Taught/Research
Do you intend to study full-time or part-time?	Full-time/Part-time
Is distance learning an option for you?	Yes/No
Does the university or college have a good reputation?	Yes/No
Are work experience or placement opportunities available?	Yes/No
Will it help you get a job? Check employment rates of graduates.	Yes/No
Is there an opportunity for further study afterwards (e.g. for a PhD)?	Yes/No
Do you meet the entry requirements?	Yes/No
What will it cost? Is any funding available?	
Is accommodation available?	Yes/No
What are the study facilities like? Are library and IT services available 24/7?	Yes/No
What support services exist for postgraduate students?	
What are the social facilities like?	

Figure 1.2: A checklist of questions to ask when choosing your programme of postgraduate study.

2

Managing work/life balance in postgraduate academic study

Dr Catherine Hayes and Sonia Bussey

Unless you are progressing from a master's degree to PhD-level study, your education up to now will have been virtually organised for you, but this experience can now be consigned to distant memory. At postgraduate level, you will definitely be expected to take responsibility for your own learning (Kell 2006). This is not to say that you have no right, as a postgraduate student, to expect good-quality educational provision. If you have an issue to raise regarding standards of provision, you should certainly do so, but it needs to be done according to the particular policies of the institution you are attending.

Above all, it is important for you to understand the difference between the nature of postgraduate study and the study that you have previously undertaken. The major issue is that you will now need to take ultimate responsibility for your work, how you manage your time and how you approach balancing the rest of your life alongside it (Birenbaum & Amdur 1999). Unlike undergraduate courses, where your teachers or facilitators would initiate areas for discussion and consideration, you will be expected to lead and develop academic debate, the basis of which may be used to inform your academic writing and submissions. This may affect your expectations of your programme and its facilitators, and also the expectations others have of you (Wisker, Robinson *et al.* 2003).

Determining the scope and nature of your research

Whichever academic institution you choose to attend, there will be a regulatory framework for your course of study. This will be open to the scrutiny of both internal and external examiners and will ensure the academic credibility of the award for which you have chosen to study. You should also note that different disciplines in the healthcare sciences will have their own characteristic research cultures. For instance, in a laboratory-based subject such as pharmacy, health and safety issues may largely determine the way research is conducted. Meanwhile, other subjects may require research of a more qualitative nature, which may involve gathering data and people's opinions (Bowling 2009).

The equipment and infrastructure needed for the research may also be an important factor in defining the area to be investigated. For example, if the work is an integral part of a larger project, its scope may be largely predetermined by the nature of the work being undertaken by the research supervisor. In this case, it will be the supervisor's responsibility to acquire the physical resources needed for the research. More qualitative research may offer students different opportunities – for instance, you may have more freedom to design and develop your own methodological approaches, while being facilitated and supported by a supervisor.

Choosing a course and where to study

If you are looking for a research-based postgraduate course, you should find out as much as possible about your future supervisor. Find about the research they are conducting themselves, where their work has been published, if they are widely respected in your field of interest and if they have an international profile. There may be information online about their research interests and background.

If you are looking for a taught programme, you should ask about the size of classes. This may influence how many seminar and tutorial groups you will have to accommodate in your academic schedule.

It's also a good idea to find out about the employment record of postgraduates from the institution. These 'graduate destination' statistics should be available from the institution or may be posted on the Unistats website (Unistats 2013). You may also want to contact potential employers to check how they would value the qualification.

Personal factors

There are also personal factors to consider. For example, you should think about the advantages of different types of location. Is there a location where you have friends or family connections? Would you prefer a big city or a smaller town? It's also worth finding out about available transport connections and opportunities for cultural activities.

Do you want to live on campus? Will this be possible at the institution? If not, you will need to check what sort of accommodation will be available. Course tuition fees will vary from place to place but some institutions may offer financial assistance. You will also need to check on availability of courses and their academic entry requirements.

Resources and support

Consider the different types of support you may need (Jacklin & Le Riche 2009). Will there be many other postgraduate students and what will be their academic background? Is there a graduate school that provides a central administrative point for graduates? What sort of English language support services will be available if you need them?

You should find out about the institution facilities. For example, is the library well stocked? Is there Internet access and will there be adequate computing facilities? It may be preferable to have a separate working space for research students.

Have you identified a supportive supervisor for your research-based programme? It is important for you to have a comfortable working relationship so, if possible, arrange to meet the supervisor before accepting a place and arrange to talk to their current research students. Also, find out whether you would be working alone or as part of a research group.

Employment prospects

You should also give careful consideration to your employment prospects on completion of your postgraduate studies. This is something you need to consider alongside your personal enthusiasm for a particular subject (unless you are in a position to be able to undertake study for study's sake at this level). Each academic institution has a department that deals with careers and employment options. It is advisable to check both with the institution you are currently attending and the one you are proposing to attend regarding transition stages between study. Both will be able to offer you help and guidance in order to make this transition as seamless as possible. Make sure you seek advice before committing to a programme of study to find out if and how the postgraduate qualification is likely to increase your chances of gaining employment afterwards.

Choosing accommodation

Mature students frequently opt to attend local (rather than far-distant) universities or colleges, on either a part-time or full-time basis. The reasons for this are often rooted in their financial commitments to home and family. Students who continue in their existing employment are also likely to want to remain close to home (NUS 2008).

For students who decide to live away from home, availability and cost of accommodation will be significant factors. In particular, availability and cost can have a significant bearing on the feasibility of living in halls of residence, and whether this will include meals provided in a dining hall or self-catering facilities. Cost and standard of provision can vary widely between educational institutions and you should visit, if possible, before making any firm decision about accommodation. The majority of educational institutions now have a designated accommodation office, which should be able to give you useful advice.

There are also particular factors to consider, regarding your personal preferences and circumstances. For instance, some universities offer single-sex accommodation, whilst in others it is mixed. If you have a partner and children to be factored into your decision-making, this will need to be considered early in order to ensure that their needs can be met too. If you think you may have special grounds for being granted financial assistance with accommodation, this ought to be discussed as soon as possible.

Remember that, once at university, you may well have to travel between campuses or to the placement opportunities provided for you. In some instances, the mileage between sites can be considerable and these journeys will need to be factored into your budget as well as your time management plans.

Childcare provision

If you have children, their welfare and happiness will be your priority, around which everything else will revolve (Wainwright & Marandet 2010). Initially, it's best to contact Student Services directly and ask as many questions as you can about any nursery or crèche facilities that are provided, the possibility of visiting to check them out, and the availability of alternative provision should you need it.

Be aware that facilities will vary immensely between different educational institutions and you will need to be absolutely certain that you are content to leave your children there during your studies, if you are to commit to a particular university or college. The Daycare Trust (Daycare Trust 2013) is a charity whose aims include promoting childcare facilities within higher education. They will be happy to provide additional advice on provision and any potential benefit entitlements.

Starting postgraduate education

You will be entering postgraduate education feeling relatively self-assured. You will have gained various undergraduate qualifications, which will have given you a sense of achievement and professional credibility. Your previous life experience will be valued by staff and colleagues. You might already be working in a healthcare organisation and you may even be a practising clinician.

Nevertheless, when seeking to progress on an academic path, there may be times when you need to acknowledge that there are gaps in your current knowledge. In order to grow, the likelihood is that you will have a significant amount to learn. Challenging the assumptions and beliefs that you accepted as an undergraduate is a normal part of postgraduate-level study. At times, this will inevitably involve a degree of self-doubt and apprehension. However, this process will enable you to develop into a person who, at the end of your postgraduate course, is capable of presenting the best evidence base for healthcare by synthesising and consolidating knowledge and stretching the boundaries of your critical thinking. As this new identity emerges, there should be opportunities for you to develop, both personally and professionally, and this process will become a tangible part of your postgraduate learning (Birenbaum & Amdur 1999).

Successful postgraduate students can think critically, read widely and write well. They can demonstrate the skills of independent thinking and the creation of knowledge, and apply these skills to the improvement of managerial-level work or, more commonly, their own continuing professional development (Kell 2006).

What are the characteristics of postgraduate study?

You will be expected to undertake wide background reading. You cannot simply rely on the material referred to in taught sessions. Reading and critically evaluating literature is the backbone of sound critical appraisal skills and will underpin your ability to demonstrate mastery of a subject.

You will also need to be able to locate and search through published literature and open it to academic scrutiny through critical evaluation. These skills are necessary to provide a basis for logical argument and discussion surrounding research evidence.

Finally, you will be expected to design your own research project, rationalise it philosophically and methodologically, justify your findings theoretically and present them (in the shape of written text and data or statistics).

What are the main issues in terms of balancing work and life?

Regular attendance and academic engagement

Regular attendance and academic engagement are pivotal to your success and will demonstrate your commitment to your postgraduate academic studies (Barlow & Fleischer 2011). If you are unwilling or unable to attend your classes and seminars on a regular basis, you need to ask yourself why. All the evidence shows that those students who engage with their academic studies do markedly better than those who regularly miss sessions.

Nevertheless, there are likely to be a few occasions when you cannot attend your sessions for unavoidable reasons and you will of course be expected to catch up with the help of colleagues. Do maintain regular contact with your academic tutors so they can help you when necessary.

If your whole motivation to attend is dwindling, address this too. It may be that counselling or personal support can help you over a difficult hurdle during your studies. Ongoing difficulties with attendance and engagement can often be resolved with support so don't hesitate to seek help as soon as possible.

Being accountable

Contingency planning is vital in order to manage the demands of academic study, particularly in the context of postgraduate teaching and learning, where most students have commitments extending far beyond their educational endeavours. Circumstances are as unique as the individual students enrolled on programmes. Illness, bereavement, relationship breakdown and caring for dependants are all part of the bigger picture, which make people human first and students second. This is not to reduce the significance of engaging with a postgraduate programme but simply to be realistic about the demands students can expect to have placed upon them (Mizrachi & Bates 2013).

You will need to foster a close relationship with your programme leader or designated personal tutor in order to manage any absence or mitigating circumstances that might affect your ability to engage with or achieve on your course. This does not mean that they will require constant detailed updates on your whereabouts, or the health of your second cousin twice removed and his paternal grandfather. The important point is to be genuine and sincere in your personal accountability. In other words, if you can't make it to a session or tutorial, let someone know so that your absence can be appropriately reported. You should also remember that your tutors and programme leaders are human and face exactly the same issues in life as you do. They are not there to judge you. They are there to support their students, and are usually more than willing to do so.

Looking after your health

Most people take their health completely for granted – until something goes wrong. However, many physical problems can be avoided or reduced by adopting a healthy lifestyle. To understand how best to preserve and protect your health and wellbeing, you need to start by acknowledging any factors that could potentially lead to ill health and also admit to yourself that it takes some willpower to guard against them.

Being and feeling healthy is more than simply being free of disease. It involves having a holistic sense of wellbeing. This depends on many factors, some of which can be controlled and others which sadly cannot (such as lack of financial security and/or a genetic predisposition to develop a particular illness). Nevertheless, developing basic strategies to stay well and feel well are important in attempting to protect your health as far as you possibly can.

Our personalities and character traits play a big part in the way we cope with stress, and our psychological reaction to stress can negatively influence our physical health through the manifestation of somatic symptoms (Gibbons 2012). Environmental and lifestyle factors also have a major influence on our health. Even if we are genetically predisposed to a particular condition, it may not necessarily develop into a physical problem. The predisposition can often be relatively well managed by making positive lifestyle choices and taking care to maintain an optimal environment.

As a student, you will need to think practically about lifestyle and environmental factors. The obvious lifestyle issues (such as smoking, alcohol intake and healthy eating) will be the same as those facing anyone else in the population. However, when working under pressure and having to manage your time and look after your health and wellbeing, it will be particularly important to keep making the right conscious choices.

If you have a specific health condition that has to be carefully managed, you will need to factor this into your decisions about where you live and where you socialise. As an adult, you will be used to managing your health and wellbeing independently in any case. But making healthy living a priority whilst you are a student can really help maximise your chances of having a productive and healthy time while studying for your postgraduate qualification.

Regular exercise

Physical activity is an excellent way of contributing to positive health and wellbeing (Vankim & Nelson 2013). Academic institutions are often well equipped with facilities such as gymnasiums and swimming pools and an array of opportunities to combine being sociable with maintaining health and wellbeing. You may never have considered taking formal exercise before, and perhaps feel that it isn't part of your persona. Yet signing up for a new sporting or leisure activity may bring with it the opportunity to meet different people, and become fitter and happier as a result. If you don't think you have time for formal exercise, simply walking or cycling to lectures (rather than driving or taking a bus) will save you money and help you stay fit and healthy.

Support systems

Each institution has its own central Students' Union – and this will be your first port of call for advice on the majority of issues.

Specific guidance and support for students with disabilities and learning difficulties (such as dyslexia and dyspraxia) is usually offered by designated teams within each educational institution. You may never have been diagnosed with a particular learning support need but academic teams and specialists in disability and dyslexia will refer you to appropriate practitioners, if they feel there is a need for intervention.

If you are not already in employment, the Careers Service will be able to offer information on applying for future professional roles. Most postgraduates will have given some consideration to the long-term 'fit' of qualification to professional opportunities. But if you are someone who has gone through relatively generic teaching programmes, this may not be the case.

Welfare issues

The vast majority of people who advise on student welfare are well-qualified professionals who have had specialist training in order to provide you with key advice on financial issues. If welfare issues are causing you problems, do address them head on and seek help with managing them straight away. Don't let these problems become something that has the potential to distract you from your studies (Galardi 2012). It is also worth noting that these issues can remain absolutely confidential, so you don't need to worry about value judgements being made about you by academic staff.

Examples of issues that you may wish to discuss with a welfare adviser, in terms of your entitlements, include:

- Student finance (e.g. student loans, tuition fees and grants)
- Current student fee status
- Fee payment problems
- Planning your budget
- Dealing with debt
- Immigration law
- International student issues
- Financial support for student parents (e.g. childcare costs)

- Postgraduate funding
- Welfare benefits and tax credits
- Disability benefits
- Study blocks that you need to pay for, due to absence
- Interrupting your studies, re-sitting exams, withdrawing or transferring
- Extenuating circumstances affecting academic performance
- Hardship funds and bursaries
- NHS funding
- Funding from trusts and charities
- Housing rights
- Council tax issues.

Considering counselling

Most people have heard of counselling but you might never have contemplated going for counselling yourself. Essentially, it is a relaxed dialogue with a practitioner, whose role is to help you explore issues that have become a barrier to your learning. This can give you a sense of perspective on life events that may be affecting your ability to progress educationally. Thinking and talking through difficulties with a neutral, objective individual can help you reflect critically on what is happening in your life. Critical reflection will not alter your circumstances but it can change the way you respond to them. You will then be able to make meaningful changes in your life, which may ultimately improve your relationships and lifestyle (Pearson 2012).

One common misconception people have is that they need to have experienced a severely traumatic event in order to benefit from counselling sessions. This is a complete myth, since counselling can always help us think of ways to move forward positively and constructively, regardless of the nature of the problem.

Emotional and psychological issues

Defining emotional resilience

'Emotional resilience' has become a buzzword in education and it is often confused with characteristics such as toughness, resistance or 'being hard-faced'. It actually means something very different, and it is an invaluable tool for students who opt to engage in postgraduate-level study. Briefly, emotional resilience is the ability to remain calm and measured in the face of adversity. In other words, it refers to how well we cope when things go pear-shaped, as they inevitably do at some point for all of us (Larned 2012).

Multiple factors can combine at any step along life's pathway to conspire against us, usually at the most inopportune of moments. This means that we all need a degree of emotional resilience in order to survive the everyday journey known as 'living'. To gain emotional resilience, we need to develop a sense of perspective. This can give us a solid grounding from which to cope when pressures (both personal and professional) mount and we still have deadlines to meet for academic work. As mentioned previously, education is an integral part of life. Like many other aspects of life, it requires us to be emotionally resilient and face up to everyday challenges.

Re-framing adversity

In this context, the term 'adversity' can be interpreted in its broadest sense. For instance, students habitually perpetuate myths about their own inability to do things. They may be troubled by self-doubt or perfectionism, seek validation, feel unable to think for themselves, or be dogged by apathy or boredom to the point of disengagement from their studies. Yet, when seen in a different light, these are simply self-fulfilling prophecies that stand in the way of personal and professional success.

If you can learn positive mental habits at this stage, it will be easier to train yourself in the art of resilience. Bouncing back from adversity is harder whilst you are in the midst of it. It's therefore better to identify potential challenges before they arise. Changing your mindset can be difficult, and hard to sustain. These positive mental habits need to become part of an overall change in attitude and reflected behaviour.

Surveying your own emotional intelligence and resilience can be a good way of establishing just how well you will cope with certain elements of study.

Belief systems

People's individual belief systems are central to their emotional resilience. Those who define their psychological being through a positive attitude and an internal locus of control, and remain optimistic in the face of adversity, contrast starkly with those who take a pessimistic view and rely on an external locus of control. This abnegation of control lends itself to the development of a negative outlook and accompanying risk of poor mental health. An individual's capacity to regulate strong emotions can, to some extent, consciously inhibit corresponding behavioural action. Controlling behavioural responses is significant, as everyone has a biologically driven temperament.

Developing coping strategies

Bearing all this in mind, it is well worth thinking about the need to develop positive mental characteristics before embarking on any educational journey. The key to resilience is being able to adopt coping strategies that allow us to bounce back from problems and negative feelings such as stress, rejection, anger, disappointment and humiliation. These strategies will ideally allow us to handle any setbacks in our experiences of teaching, learning and assessment.

It is also worth remembering that resilience can be acquired, like any other skill, and initially it is not easy. Life in itself necessitates a degree of resilience in terms of everything that is thrown at us, which might explain why younger people usually have less emotional resilience than those who are mature. Also, some people who have had few adverse impacts in their lives may have a correspondingly low degree of emotional resilience, simply because they have never needed it.

The skills and tools we need to harbour emotional resilience are free. They include talking through problems with friends, learning how to be reflexive (not just reflective), and taking care of our general health and wellbeing by adopting a healthy lifestyle. However, the most fundamental point to remember is that we are all human. Feeling negative emotion is normal, and at any stage of study you only fail when you give up and you don't learn from the experience. Life goes on, regardless of how disappointed we are. This may sometimes be hard to believe but it is reassuringly true.

This chapter has provided a very brief insight into how studying can become an integrated part of daily life, rather than something that has to be tackled in abstraction. There are numerous sources of support as you make the transition from either the workplace or another educational institution into academic study at postgraduate level. Don't be afraid to ask for help in terms of the decisions you are making or for information on how previous students have experienced programmes of study that you might be considering. This can be a valuable way of making new connections and finding out about the details of postgraduate experience that are important considerations for your everyday life but might not necessarily be part of an institutional prospectus. From a practical point of view, this type of information-gathering can be as valuable as researching the academic programme you might wish to study.

3

Postgraduate-level study skills

Shelagh Keogh

It is assumed that a student undertaking a master's degree course has either been formally accredited with an undergraduate degree or has the experience and skills expected of a successful undergraduate degree graduate. Mastering a skill once does not mean that it is embedded forever; all skills must be practiced and continuously updated. A postgraduate student will therefore need to master all the skills mastered by an undergraduate student, plus some additional elements.

Choosing what to read

If you are just starting out on your journey to understand a new subject you can use certain techniques to help you progress. In undertaking postgraduate study, one of your aims will be to acquire knowledge. This does not happen automatically but requires a strategic approach to learning. For instance, you can pick up a journal article and read it but this will not necessarily result in understanding the paper or the subject being discussed.

Firstly, you should choose the paper carefully. Begin by identifying the relevant journals in your subject area. Your subject librarians will have already carried out this search. You can access this information via your tutors, in the reading lists they give you, or you can explore for yourself by using one of the many free websites available for the purpose, such as http://eigenfactor.org/.

Once you have found your journal, you need to search for the appropriate articles; this is both an art and a science. The more you know about the subject, the easier it is to locate the relevant material. To search for articles of interest, you will need to enter key words or authors' names. As you search and read various articles, you will soon realise that there are many possible keywords related to the subject you are trying to find. It is a good idea to keep a record of the keywords you use, and those that give you the greatest number of 'hits'. There are various software packages available to help you manage your searches/citations, such as Endnote, which is available in Microsoft Word. At the end of your search, you should have identified most of the key journals, key authors, current issues and/or areas of interest in your subject.

Getting the most out of your reading

Having located the articles, you can read them and develop your knowledge and understanding. However, you cannot really engage with academic papers in the same way as you might read a magazine or journal article. Again, you need to employ strategies to get the most out of them. Firstly, try reading the article and then answering the following questions:

1. What is the focus of the paper?

2. Why is this important to your subject area?

3. What was being measured in the research?

4. What did the research prove or disprove?

5. What was the conclusion of the paper?

6. Do you agree with the author or authors? If yes or no, why?

To capture the knowledge:

- Try to summarise the paper in two to four sentences.
- List the authors' main assumptions, the techniques they used, their results and their conclusions.
- Make brief notes on how you would change or improve on their work if you were carrying out the research yourself.

Edward de Bono (De Bono 1999, De Bono & Zimbalist 2010) is a guru in thinking and has published many books that help people use their minds more effectively. The way our minds work can inhibit our progress, unless we train ourselves to use them well. Our minds are always ready to respond to the world around us, and our defence mechanisms (the 'flight or flight' response) keep us safe. This part of the brain is immediate and instinctive. But when engaging with study we need to use the logical element. This part of the brain requires time. We need to process our thoughts and then embed them in our deep memories, so that we can access the knowledge when we need to connect it to other thoughts in the future.

Here is another useful technique (based on the work of Edward de Bono) that will help you engage more fully with a subject. Once you have read a paper or book, list:

- All the positives
- All the negatives
- All the interesting items that are neither positive nor negative but may become one or the other
- All the alternative approaches to the techniques, tools and/or approaches used in the paper, book or article
- All the constraints, such as time, money and skills, that would affect this area of interest

Independent study skills

Achievement of knowledge requires a student to set themselves personal standards. In postgraduate study there is greater emphasis on independent study and there are a number of independent learning skills that you can develop. Some of these skills are considered below.

Having the freedom to set your own agenda for the day requires a disciplined approach. Some postgraduate degree pathways may incorporate minimal contact time, but, for every hour of contact time with your tutors, you should set aside at least a further two hours of independent learning time.

To help you achieve this, you might want to consider where you learn best. You should note that this is not necessarily the same as your favourite place. The best place to learn may be in a particular venue – perhaps the library, in an open access area or at home. But ask yourself whether that is because it is most pleasant or because it is where you are likely to produce a lot of work. You also need to consider when is the best time to study – in the morning, afternoon or late at night. Ask yourself when you are likely to learn most effectively. As you probably know, it is possible to spend a long time studying but not really get much out of a particular session, so it is a good idea to set objectives for each study period.

We all have access to formal and informal resources that can assist us in our study. The formal ones will be advertised by your educational institution, and include things like study skills sessions. There may also be professional bodies, interest groups on the Internet and study groups that you have formed with other students. When setting your study agenda, think about the ways in which these resources can help you achieve your objectives.

We all know that good time management is needed for any successful endeavour. But it is still a challenge to apply this knowledge in order to ensure good working practices. We do not have limitless time (just as we do not have limitless money) but we are usually better at managing our money than our time. However, good time management really is the key to being able to cope and develop in postgraduate education. There are many well-known time management techniques and some of the most effective ones are listed below:

- Set aside a length of time for study, say 4 hours
- Break this down into 15-minute periods
- Write against each period what you are going to achieve in that 15 minutes.

At the bottom of the page, note whether or not you have been effective in this study period; you may have been too ambitious or not ambitious enough. Writing this note allows you to reflect on your performance and make improvements for subsequent sessions.

Recording your efforts

Draw up a study sheet as shown in the sample below.

Study objective: Write a chapter in my dissertation

Deliverable at end of study period: A draft dissertation chapter [or some concrete and measurable achievement]

Date: 15.01.14   **Start time**: 09.00   **End time**: 13.00   **Duration**: 4 hours

Period	Achievement (complete as you go)
09.00–09.15	Set out chapter structure
09.15–09.30	Write 500 words, Section One of chapter
09.15–09.30	
09.30–09.45	
09.45–10.00 etc	

Commentary

Did you achieve your objective? ....

On a scale of 1 to 10 (with 10 being objective fully achieved), how would you score yourself? ....

Were you too ambitious? ....

Were you not ambitious enough? ....

Most students today use their phones for every kind of activity, including managing their time. There are good time trackers that allow you to record your activities and send you a report at set intervals on how you have used your time. Use a search engine to look up time tracker apps.

Being organised and managing your time

Even if you are not the most organised person in the world, it's worth learning to allocate time slots to your teaching and learning activities so that you can get a realistic idea of where the rest of your life needs to be adjusted while you are undertaking your studies. Above all, stay positive and remember why you have opted to take your course of study. All your hard work will be worthwhile once you have achieved your qualification. Establishing what you want to achieve on a practical level upon completion of your studies can sometimes help you work out your starting point and come to terms with the academic journey you are embarking upon.

You will have to submit various academic assignments to different tutors throughout your course. You therefore need to structure your study to ensure that you meet the relevant delivery dates. There may be occasions when two are due on the same day, which means prioritising the one that has to be completed first. You may wish to keep this information in a visible place, say on a wall. You can of course keep it on your phone or on a computer but will you look at it if it is not visible on a day-to-day basis? You should not consider the deadline as your submission date; this is the very last time you can submit, rather than the only time. Missing a deadline can mean failing a module or subject. Depending on your course regulations, you may not get the opportunity to retake the subject again, which could mean failing your whole course.

To avoid this, it's a good idea to chart out specific time slots in which certain things can be achieved. Being busy and being productive are two different things; and being genuinely productive can make a significant difference to overall achievement. Most people can find or plan half an hour extra in order to get things done. For example, you could get up an hour earlier or you could designate part of each day (which is currently spent on something unproductive) as time to be spent on some academic contribution to your studies. It might be something as straightforward as selecting and retrieving relevant literature, rather than just surfing the Internet for half an hour a day. Or you could sacrifice watching a half-hour television programme and instead dedicate that time to critical appraisal of your work to date. Over an academic year, this could contribute a significant amount to the time you are able to spend on your academic work. Once these time slots are habitually allocated to work, it will become second nature.

Keep an area at home where you can study and get into the habit of doing half an hour's work whenever you have time to do so. If you have a designated room or space, you won't need to set up a working area each time, before you can actually get down to studying.

You should also try to allocate a set length of time to engage with your studies so that you can be focused on your work, rather than drifting aimlessly through a time slot which is either too long to maintain your concentration or too short to allow you to settle into working.

Even if you are not a 'list person', it's well worth making a 'to do' list that is achievable and realistic so that you can monitor your progress through your studies. You will also find that scheduling your work will mean that you are much more likely to undertake it. If you have a large piece of work that you feel daunted by, try to break it down into more manageable chunks that you can tackle systematically. Another good tip is that you should always do the most difficult part first – this way you can look forward to the completion of your work with a sense of optimism.

If you are committing to other activities with colleagues, family and friends, learn to prioritise what is important to you (Grund, Brassler *et al.* 2013). See also whether you can set some personal goals with an identifiable timeline, which you can follow in order to map out your achievement by a particular date. Your ability to be flexible is paramount in order to build resilience so that you can cope when things go wrong. Being free to reorganise your own time at short notice will allow you to stay in control and keep in mind why you originally wanted to undertake your course of study as part of your personal long-term goals.

If you are a full-time student you should treat study just as you would a full-time job. From the beginning of your course, set aside the time from 09.00 to 17.00 each day, taking breaks for lunch, coffee, and so on. Then you can use the evenings and weekends for social and domestic activities. Most students have a tendency to wait until they are given deadlines by their tutors for assessments or academic assignments; good students set their own deadlines and this disciplined approach will be really useful for your future employment.

Making the most of opportunities

One of the main purposes of a university is research, which is directed by members of the academic staff. There will be numerous opportunities while you are at university to attend seminars where researchers will present their studies. It is usual to invite students to attend these sessions. If you have not had an invitation, ask your tutor for the published schedule.

Every time an academic is made a professor they give professorial lectures. These can be very engaging and will demonstrate the level of achievement you are aiming for in your research. Professorial lectures are usually advertised and open for you to attend, although you may have to book a place.

Many professional bodies hold free seminars with employers in different regions of the country. Check out the professional body for your subject area to see if they have advertised any such seminars, or if they are available through teleconferencing.

Your tutors will give you reading lists at the beginning of the course, and you should decide which books you need to buy, and which ones you can obtain through the library. Some books will be available electronically, while some will be available to purchase second-hand through bookshops (both online and on-campus). You should purchase or borrow books early in the course when you are under less pressure.

Taking responsibility and prioritising tasks

Are you someone who drives their own learning or are you a passenger on your educational journey? As we pointed out at the beginning of this chapter, postgraduate study requires you to be an autonomous practitioner. In higher education, students are expected to understand what is required of them and to work out their own strategies to enable them to achieve their objectives. Successful postgraduate students don't wait for others to start the process; they set their own timetable and objectives.

Once you realise that your destiny lies in your own hands, it is much easier to use the resources available to achieve your aims. You will be under a lot of pressure, and you will need to prioritise your tasks according to their relative urgency. It is also up to you to decide how much time to spend on each task. You will want to carry out each assignment to the best of your ability, while remembering that perfection is not usually achievable.

The following questions will help you prioritise and plan your work:

- Can you make a list of activities or tasks that you need to complete?
- What is the expected output from each task? (All tasks should have measurable and deliverable outputs. If not, they are probably steps within other tasks.)
- What would happen if this task were not completed?
- Does this task need to be completed before another task can begin?
- What is the secondary task that needs the outputs of this task?
- How good does the output of this task have to be?
- What resources are needed to complete this task?
- Do you have full access to the resources required?

- How long will it take to complete this task?
- Where would be the most *productive* place to work in order to complete this task?

Asking these questions will help you understand and prioritise the tasks you need to carry out.

Being creative and innovative

There is no magic tool or technique that enables students to be creative and innovative, but you can train yourself to make the most of your mind and other people's minds. If you go to a design studio and compare it to a medical lab, you will see immediately that they are very different in their look and feel. The design studio may be full of colour and disorder, but out of this disorder will come many new ways to do things. Everywhere you turn, there will be things that inspire you to move away from your normal automatic thinking patterns and explore other ways of applying knowledge. Working with others will also help you to be creative and innovative. Sharing and challenging each other's knowledge base helps generate new knowledge, but you have to be open to sharing knowledge in the first place.

When a student graduates and has to go into the world of work, they rarely find a perfect atmosphere in which to make decisions calmly and clearly. If decisions have to be made, it is usually because there is an urgent need to do so. This is why you are often challenged in assignments to answer questions where the answers are not immediately obvious. Developing these skills requires you to understand the decision-making or problem-solving process. We all make decisions every day but most of them are not life-changing so our habitual, automatic thinking processes can usually deal with them.

When you are under pressure to make a decision, it is best to use a framework to arrive at your answers. Some very good decision-making frameworks have been worked out by philosophers and politicians. An interesting article by Savio and Nikolopoulos (2013) makes some useful points on this subject.

Complex situations usually require several decisions to be made, and many different responses could be given to each of these decisions. Every response can affect different people in many ways. Once we have made a decision, we do not know exactly how people will respond to it. The complex nature of our world means that sometimes we don't even find out what impact our actions have had after the event. Yet, even though we do not always see the results, they can be far reaching. An interesting leadership framework tool is the Cynefin framework, formulated by Snowden and Boone (2007). This framework, like others, sets out a series of questions to apply a situation. Again this aid can help you understand a situation or subject more deeply. (For more on frameworks, see below.)

Developing yourself professionally

No one is more interested in you than yourself. We spend much of our lives at work so we should try to get the best out of ourselves as we pass through life. Regardless of whether or not your programme of study is associated with a particular professional body, you should therefore approach your studies and placements in a professional manner. To be a professional is to be someone who:

- Continually assesses their strengths and weaknesses and does not wait for an event such as an annual appraisal to do so
- Understands what skills they need to carry out activities in their profession
- Knows how to improve the weaknesses in their skill set
- Embraces opportunities to enhance their skills, without undertaking work that they are not competent to do
- Ensures that they keep up to date with the latest thinking in their profession
- Contributes to the debates within their profession.

To achieve all this, we need to set time aside for reflection. The ultimate praise anyone can give professionals is that they are reflective practitioners – that is, people who continuously learn from experience.

You can use frameworks to help you reflect on your skills, and there will probably be several available for your use from your professional body's website. At some point during your studies, you will probably be asked to present a professional development assessment, usually known as a Professional Development Plan (PDP). Most PDP frameworks cover the same areas:

- Setting goals to achieve your objectives
- Listing activities required to achieve the objectives
- Setting deadlines for your goals and milestones for your activities
- Reflecting at the milestones as to whether the goals are still relevant and whether the activities are still appropriate to achieve the objectives
- Listing the resources you will need to achieve your goals and objectives.

Developing yourself professionally and undergoing personal reflection can be hard at times. Do not underestimate how long each task will take or how difficult it may be. The best way to work out a sensible plan is to talk it over with someone else. However, before you can talk about your plan to another person, you need to establish an open, trusting relationship. Putting your weaknesses down on paper is like opening up your hidden self to others – even if you are the only one who will read the whole document.

Communicating

In all higher education courses, you need to communicate your study findings with others. This could take many different forms, including writing, presentations, posters, and contributions at conferences.

When starting a new course, you should reflect on how you have previously communicated in your studies and whether you have developed good or bad habits. In the first few weeks of your course, there will be fewer demands on your time than can be expected later on. This is therefore a good time to revisit good practice on communication skills, and there are many helpful study guides available

One common mistake is not planning written assignments sufficiently well. Essays often start well, then drift off and then become more focused towards the end; or they fail to introduce or conclude the work adequately. Both problems are usually the result of not spending enough time planning and considering how you are going to communicate your work to others.

You should always plan out your essay before starting to write it. Begin with the title at the top, then break it down into sub-headings, bearing in mind what your tutor will be expecting you to cover in your response. If you are finding this difficult, it is probably best to read your assessment brief again, to ensure that you understand what is expected of you. Once you have an overall structure for your response to the question, it will be far easier to fill in the individual sections, rather than trying to complete the whole assignment in one go.

When you have completed your essay, set it aside for at least 24 hours, and then review your response against the question set, not forgetting to spell check and grammar check throughout. Of course, giving yourself time at the end of an assessment to check the quality of your submission will require good time management.

If you are writing an examination, you won't have the luxury of 24 hours before checking the quality but it is equally important to plan. You should allow some time after answering each question to ensure that you have been focused in your response. At the start of the examination, you should divide up the time for each question according to the points allocated to it, while remembering to allow time for reading and checking the quality of your answers.

Working with others

The notion of collaborative and social learning may not immediately spring to mind when enrolling for a postgraduate programme of study. However, collaborative working has many benefits at postgraduate level (Yadegaridehkordi, Iahad, *et al.* 2013), which are briefly summarised below:

1. The process of collaboration can help you open your work up for commentary. This prevents writing papers from becoming a solitary activity and also enables you to understand that writing can be much improved through feedback from a critical friend. This is particularly useful prior to submitting any piece of work for formal peer review.

2. Particularly for non-taught postgraduate level study, focusing and writing work for a specific academic audience through a particular style of academic discourse can initially present quite a challenge for students. The opportunity to work collaboratively can help you meet this challenge.

3. Collaborative working is also useful because it creates a degree of shared expectation and anticipation during an academic journey. Through sharing your experience of individual teaching and learning processes, you will find it easier to reflect upon your academic progress.

4. Collaboration affords you the opportunity to engage with others and to demonstrate your developing sense of mastery over an aspect of study. This not only permits a degree of self-reflection; it also engenders a desire to improve and understand the art of communicating complex information to a wide range of audiences.

Working with others is a challenge and requires attention, just like other aspects of your studies. In the real world I cannot think of any occupation that doesn't require some degree of co-operation. When you first start working with others on group assessments, it is best to give yourself a little time to think about how 'I' am going to get the best out of others and out of myself. One of the most common issues is that one or two members of the group do not contribute as much as others, or the quality of their work is not as high as the work of others.

If one member of the group is not contributing as much, start by asking yourself whether the rest of the group (including you) are allowing them to contribute. Some people are really good in group discussion, while others are more reticent but still have some very valuable views to contribute if given the time and space to do so.

Sometimes it happens that work has been allocated at the start of the group interaction but the skills of individuals have not been taken into consideration and hence some may not have the tools they need to carry out the work. To avoid this problem arising, it's a good idea to carry out a skills audit at the first meeting of the group. You should identify what skills are needed for the assignment, then map these out on a grid and ask each person to rate themselves for each skill. It may be that no member possesses certain skills, in which case the group may need to develop a strategy to overcome this.

If a member of the group produces work that is not considered to be of the required quality, they may need help in understanding the group's expectations; this may not have been clear when the work was being allocated. The group should also check the quality of all the work contributed while there is still time to correct any defects.

Bearing all these points in mind, you may wish to develop a group code of conduct. This document should be used to guide expectations and to prevent problems arising. Each code included in the document should be followed by the reason for its inclusion. The document should also be given sufficient weight to ensure that group members will taken it into consideration and understand the consequences should they not adhere to it. An example of such a code is given on page 37

Conclusion

Having signed up for a master's course, you should be aware that your studies will be student-centred and not tutor-led. You should already have a well-developed skill set from your previous study and should thus be able to drive your own learning forward. We often look to others when we find things difficult but in reality our destiny is in our own hands. The more we learn, the more enjoyable and exciting life becomes.

Finally here is a useful checklist, which you can use to check the quality of your work. Having produced an assignment, ask yourself these questions:

What would my best friend think of this assignment submission?

Would I be proud to show my mother or father my submission?

Would I be proud to have this submission published online or in print?

Sample group code of conduct

Code 1

Each member of the group agrees to attend all group meetings. Missing one session will mean a yellow card (warning) is held against their name on the records. Missing two meetings will mean that their attendance and commitment to the group is discussed by the others at the meeting and action is taken accordingly. The action might mean that the offending member of the group has to buy each of the other group members a drink, or if it is more serious the group member will be reported to the course or study tutor.

Reason for the code: To ensure efficiency in communication and sharing of knowledge

Code 2:

Each member of the group will format their findings in accordance with the group's corporate style:

- Font - Times New Roman
- Pitch – 11
- Margins – Word definition of normal
- Headings – Word definition of 'Header 2'

Reason for the code: To ensure efficiency when merging work together at the final group meeting.

Final Code:

If any member of the group does not adhere to the group codes, action will be taken as in Code 1 above.

4

Work-based learning in postgraduate health curricula

Dr Catherine Hayes

In many postgraduate programmes (especially those associated with a particular professional area), there is often a work-based learning component. The way this is organised depends on the programme in question. In some programmes, students are expected to demonstrate their achievement of particular competencies. In others, students are required to undertake a specific work-based project. This chapter aims to explore the key issues around work-based learning, some of which may not apply to your particular programme.

What are the characteristics of work-based learning?

It is difficult to provide one overarching definition for work-based learning, due to the vast variation in the way educational and organisational providers design their courses (Nikolova et al. 2014). This type of learning is also sometimes known as 'experiential learning', 'situated learning' and 'work-based practice learning'. There may be subtle differences in execution but, in the majority of cases, you will be able to individualise your work-based learning experience (Park et al. 2014). You can often negotiate particular learning outcomes for what you plan to achieve in practice. As well as developing particular clinical skills, it is important to remember that you also need to apply theoretical perspectives to practice. Reflecting on your practice and skill development is an important part of this process (Thomas et al. 2014). Practical learning is often associated with the reality of human interaction, which reflects real life in the workplace (McMenamin et al. 2014). At postgraduate level, work-based learning helps you develop your higher-order critical thinking skills. This will equip you to undertake complex clinical decision-making processes at the front line of patient care. Work-based learning requires students to demonstrate autonomy, intrinsic motivation and active engagement in order to have the greatest impact on the learning experience.

Situated learning experience (or learning 'in situ') helps students develop their ability to lead, to manage change and to ensure quality. These are all features of a high-quality workforce. This type of learning is based on the seminal work of Lave and Wenger (1991), extended most recently by Ainley and Rainbird (2014). Research in this field continues to acknowledge the role of 'communities of practice' in the context of teaching and learning and the significance of learning from those with expertise. Essentially, situated learning is problem-based but solution-focused. In other words, students learn in the context of real-life healthcare provision to manage contingency, assess risk and make complex decisions that affect the lives of patients and their families and carers.

Fitness to practise

Fitness to practise is a concept that underpins the professional ethos of healthcare delivery in the UK. This transcends any knowledge and skill base and is a values system focused on how individual attitudes are translated into professional behaviour at the front line of patient care. Professionalism is a topic that has been intensely debated by academics in recent years, especially in relation to how it ought to be assessed in practice. Anyone involved in work-based learning needs to keep 'fitness to practise' requirements in mind. They are fundamental to your conduct, your professionalism and the overall impact that your presence has in the working environment.

Your 'fitness to practise' will be monitored:

- Prior to academic or clinical staff signing any 'Good Health and Character Declarations' required by professional regulatory bodies before you apply for registration with a professional body upon completion of your studies
- Where there is concern in relation to any aspect of your conduct, your health or ability
- If you have, or if you are alleged to have, breached the regulations of the university, the department or other regulatory professional body
- If you have been suspended or excluded from practice for any reason
- If academic misconduct has been proven in any context
- If you demonstrate unprofessional behaviour in a university, clinical or external environment (e.g. misuse of the Internet and social networking sites, breach of patient/client confidentiality, failure to maintain appropriate professional or sexual boundaries, engaging in unlawful discrimination)
- If you fail to report any criminal conviction or caution (this includes failure to disclose any changes to your character status since commencement of the programme)

- If you are required to attend Occupational Health Services (e.g. if you have undertaken a leave of absence that requires a health assessment to ascertain your fitness to return to your studies)
- If you fail to recognise the limits of your own abilities, or demonstrate a lack of insight into health concerns that is likely to put others at risk
- If you are dishonest with an intention to deceive (e.g. forging your mentor's or tutor's name on clinical assessments or documentation, fraudulently presenting documentation or misrepresenting your qualifications)
- If you fail to adhere to postgraduate programme requirements (e.g. non-compliance with vaccinations, non-attendance at mandatory training sessions, failure to consistently submit programme documentation/placement assessment documentation in a timely manner)
- If you are in debt to the educational institution you are studying with
- If you do not consistently engage with the programme and its associated work-based learning opportunities, and you have failed to make regular contact with your supervisor regarding your progress.

Organisational strategies that promote work-based learning

In recent years, organisations have emphasised the importance of:

- Multi-disciplinary teamwork

- Interprofessional learning

- Continuing professional development

- Creativity and innovation in assessment

- Emergent simulation technology.

Multi-disciplinary teamwork

Collaborative, co-operative teamwork lies at the heart of effective healthcare education in the context of compassionate patient-centred care. It requires you to recognise your own 'niche' and understand where it fits in relation to the work of others, with regard to providing reliable and competent care (Hill & Hulya 2014).

Interprofessional learning

Interprofessional learning between different healthcare disciplines is now an integral part of patient-centred care and is regarded as a focal point in curriculum development (Alinier *et al.* 2014). It not only affords you the chance to examine the scope of practice of other healthcare practitioners; more valuably it gives you the opportunity to reflect on your own contribution.

Continuing professional development (CPD)

CPD is now the norm, rather than something that only the most motivated healthcare practitioners engage with (Chou *et al.* 2014). You will need to consider this, and differentiate between those aspects of CPD that are compulsory and those that you proactively choose to do because you are most interested in them and find them particularly useful.

Creativity and innovation in assessment

Creativity and innovation in assessment means allowing teaching and learning to drive assessment processes, and enabling students to negotiate how they will fulfil particular learning outcomes (Ellis 2014). Achieving these outcomes usually requires students to integrate case-based scenarios and action learning sets, which are structured activities that allow student groups to be supported through projects that can have an impact on practice. These activities are commonly referred to as 'applied practice projects' (where access to expert facilitation helps to drive the process of teaching and learning). They are ideal in the context of workplace learning.

Emergent simulation technology

Work-based learning has developed at an exponential rate through the use of interactive simulation technology. This often prompts comparisons with the aviation industry, where staff members also need to be trained in high-risk processes and procedures using simulation (Eunjung & Reeves 2014).

Tri-partite learning

Tri-partite learning involves learning experiences being deliberately linked to the strategic needs of employing organisations, where teaching, learning and assessment mechanisms can be tailored to individual students and their employers (McClatchey & Bridges 2014). To implement this approach, it would be wise to arrange a formal meeting with your employer to ensure that you have a shared vision of your learning needs, which can be effectively communicated to your educational provider.

All these strategies are highly dependent on the existence of good organisational infrastructure. They also rely on your capacity to engage in a degree of critical reflection on the clinical experience you have gained and consider how this will be developed in the future.

Acknowledging the difference between competence and proficiency

Academics frequently debate the difference between competence and proficiency and how this ought to be expressed in postgraduate assessment provision (Xiao, Wang & Ferguson 2014). There is one major point to understand here – competence is an all-or-nothing phenomenon; you are either competent or you aren't. The very fact that you are contemplating postgraduate healthcare study will usually mean that you have already achieved competence in a preliminary healthcare degree. Postgraduate study that assesses the development of the skills you have gained at undergraduate level is not checking your competence; it is evaluating your proficiency and your capacity for professional development. This is worth thinking about, particularly in relation to your own reflection on practice, as it can help you identify your inherent strengths and weaknesses and consider how to continually improve your individual contribution to patient-centred care.

Assessment in work-based learning

Assessment in work-based learning often involves producing a portfolio of evidence that incorporates critical self-reflection and some action research (in other words, investigating and/or changing an aspect of clinical practice or provision).

The standards of assessment that you are likely to have to work to usually require you to:

1. Underpin clinical practice with an academic knowledge of the relevant clinical area

2. Benchmark your pre-existing knowledge alongside that of your peer group, in terms of how much you need to develop (Moriber *et al.* 2014).

It is sometimes easy to lose sight of the fact that healthcare curricula are developed with the intention of improving patient-centred care. Incorporating practical learning into educational curricula can be an important element in institutional improvement agendas. The central message here is to be realistic and methodologically robust. Evidence-based decision-making and critical reflection on your own performance will be your most vital tools. Think of assessment in its simplest terms as a tangible means of measuring what you have learned.

It is useful for you to consider what stage of learning you have reached and what you hope to achieve. Preparing yourself for maximum engagement with the workplace could, for example, entail asking yourself some critical questions, such as:

1. Do you understand the specific type of healthcare provided by the practice area in which you are being placed?

2. Do you understand how the infrastructure works in this practice area?

3. How would you measure professionalism there? For instance, who do you need to listen to and what do you need to reflect on?

4. Can you see the need to foster collaborative working with others?

5. Are you aware of the concept of knowledge transfer?

6. Accountability in healthcare is a fundamental element of healthcare provision – are you aware of your area of accountability in the context of this placement?

7. Discipline-specific knowledge of your field of practice is pivotal to the success of your work – what does your professional regulatory body recommend in terms of work-based experiential learning beyond your initial qualification?

8. How are you managing your own expectations in relation to the work-based learning experience you are being given?

In lifelong learning, practical experience in a specific context is vital to the acquisition of new knowledge and skills. Central to the success of this type of learning is the question of how best you will be supported in practice. Social interaction in the workplace serves to position people in a social framework with which they can readily identify and relate. This increases their capacity to solve problems and make a useful contribution through collaboration with other members of the team.

Workplace culture is therefore central to your overall learning experience. Without mutual regard, equity and a sense of personal value, your gains from experiential learning will be negligible. In the workplace, people naturally develop adaptive strategies that permit the bypassing of questions and problems, and point to ready solutions. You will find it extremely helpful to evaluate these solutions, and reflect upon them.

Informal learning is a process of reconstructing and reinterpreting practice to form the basis of knowledge. Thus, learning and work can combine to form a seamless whole.

Mentorship in postgraduate work-based learning

In the context of postgraduate learning, the mentorship relationship will be framed by:

1. The extent of the pre-existing knowledge, skills and experience that you bring to the postgraduate programme

2. How the teaching and learning process from your placements drives the process of assessment

3. Whether work-based learners are integrated into the workforce in the practice area or they are additional to the institutional workforce.

The specific context of the mentoring relationship both individualises the experience and makes the process more complex. In different healthcare practice areas, there may be distinct differences in the way knowledge, skills and professional behaviours are developed. It is not easy to translate all this into a mutually understood relationship that encompasses all these aspects of learning. However, this shared understanding of the process of mentorship can ultimately facilitate learning and ensure the longevity of the professional relationship between mentor and student (Kostovich, Saban & Collins 2010). This context will also ultimately dictate fundamental aspects of the process of mentorship which are pivotal to a progressive and mutually satisfying relationship for both mentor and mentee (Jefferies & Skidmore 2010).

- The major aspects to consider are:
- How you and your mentor manage time
- How challenging behaviour can be effectively managed without conflict
- How the development of strong interpersonal and communication skills can enhance your relationship with your mentor during your studies
- How effective feedback mechanisms can be developed and realistically maintained
- How the process can be documented and recorded appropriately within the guidelines of professional regulatory bodies such as the Nursing and Midwifery Council (NMC) or those professional bodies governed by the Health Care Professions Council (HCPC).

Issues like these underpin the philosophy of mentorship, which recognises the various social and professional transitions you and your mentor undergo (Kadivar 2010). The role of the mentor should gradually change according to your professional progress. For instance, at the beginning of the relationship, you are likely to be more dependent upon your mentor. This will necessitate regular meetings and feedback and a higher degree of commitment from both of you than at a later stage in the relationship, when you (the student) will have established a high degree of professional autonomy and will be working independently. This process will affect the way the relationship works and changes over time, and you will need to agree how best this should operate. In its most basic form, it is possible to break the role of the mentor into that of an organiser and a communicator (Bulut, H., Hisar, F. & Demir, S.G. 2010).

The philosophy of the mentoring relationship

What is common and fundamental to every mentoring relationship is the philosophy of social constructivism. Social constructivism underlies not only the teaching and learning mechanisms involved in skill acquisition but also the motivation to achieve competence and proficiency. A key theorist in this discipline was Lev Vygotsky, who proposed that people learn through social experience and interaction (Vygotsky 1978). As a postgraduate student, this is particularly relevant to the subject of mentorship, and the essential points to remember are that:

- Learning and development remain embedded and social, collaborative activities.
- Teaching and learning activities should be reality-based and applicable to the real world, and – wherever possible – linked to patients and the context-specific environments in which care is provided.
- Learning extends to your social background and your interaction with life and the external world to date. All these interactions subsequently form the basis of your experience as someone learning in the context of healthcare provision.

Regardless of your particular academic discipline, the concepts of connection and separation are central to the development of your knowledge and understanding and the value judgements you use to underpin your clinical professional practice. In essence:

- Separate behaviour is the notion of objectivity and formalisation of ideas. Taking this approach, the mentor will attempt to apply logic to the situation and be relatively closed to the exploration of issues beyond the parameters of the mentorship arrangement.
- Connected behaviour is a subjective, empathic approach in which the mentor accepts that the personal attributes of a mentee underpin their professional behaviour. By aiming to listen and ask questions, a greater understanding of the student's stance can be achieved.
- Constructed behaviour is a holistic approach whereby the mentor can effectively utilise both separate and connected approaches, depending on the specific context of the interaction. Constructed behaviour gives the mentor a flexible and responsive approach, which offers logic alongside understanding so that mentees are better able to socially construct meaning around their experience.

Completing documentation

The governance and regulation of the mentorship relationship is fundamental to the whole process, and each professional regulatory body within the health sciences may have its own specific requirements for formal mentorship. If there is no formalised process of mentorship, then – at a minimum – the following dual signed documentation should exist:

Mentor	Mentee
Contractual organisations for the mentoring relationship*	
Time-keeping and attendance	
Managing the session	Preparing for the session
Ensuring the quality of support	Establishing learning needs and objectives
Monitoring the effectiveness of the relationship	Applying learning from the session
Giving feedback	Receiving feedback
Monitoring ethical and professional issues	Self-awareness in pastoral issues
Keeping additional notes, as required	
Reflection on and evaluation of the mentorship programme	

* This refers to any service level agreements between the educational institution and an external mentorship provider. For example, you might be undertaking an academic programme of study at university but this might include work experience in industrial chemistry at a neighbouring pharmaceutical institution. The university and the pharmaceutical institution will therefore have a service level agreement clarifying the terms and conditions of the arrangement.

Notes should be succinct and legible, and a copy of each set of notes should be retained by both the mentor and mentee, with due regard for confidentiality in the process (NMC 2010). These are usually very brief notes, which serve as a basic outline and reminder for both mentor and mentee of the session content. The notes are signed by both parties at the end of each meeting, and both keep a copy for their records.

Giving and receiving feedback

In the context of mentorship, giving and receiving feedback can be used to develop better relationships (Lave & Wenger 1991). Unfortunately, the term 'feedback' has acquired negative connotations because it is often used as a euphemism for being able to personally criticise someone in their chosen area of practice. Contrary to this, in the context of the mentoring relationship, feedback should be used to actively encourage both personal motivation and the core skills of professional development. By this stage of a mentee's career, the formalised systems of appraisal and professional development pathway planning will probably be an integral part of their role.

From a psychological perspective, Maslow (1954) was the first to emphasise the concept of motivation and explicitly link this to productivity and psychological wellbeing in the workplace. Acknowledging and recognising a job well done is a fundamental motivator for future development and progression. Each individual will have a preferred mechanism for receiving praise. Whereas some mentees prefer their motivation to continue working hard to come from a basic identification of where they have best achieved and an acknowledgement of it, others may prefer a more explicitly constructed explanation of how they can perform to an even higher level next time.

Professional development

Maximising every mentee's opportunity to reach their full potential is the fundamental role of every mentor, regardless of the context of the mentoring relationship. Within an organisational hierarchy, it is essential to acknowlege that all employees have room to improve. In this way, everyone can feel free to build on their pre-existing achievements and develop further within a safe environment. This ethos underpins effective professional development (Nash & Scammell 2009).

A mentor may also identify and address a need for a mentee to significantly improve a core proficiency within their professional role (Marshall & Gordon 2010). In this situation, the term 'underperforming' may be used, and this is where the language of 'negative feedback' can begin. Nevertheless, this type of feedback can become a hugely positive contribution to a mentee's personal and professional development when it is carried out in a sensitive, non-confrontational fashion. It can be particularly effective if the mentee, within the context of their peer group, is enabled to identify the weakness themselves. They can subsequently use this as a focus for improvement – without feeling pre-judged in the situation.

Essentially, feedback should be a two-way communication process about someone's performance, which allows the mentee sufficient time and space for self-reflection. The mentor may be tempted to move straight into their general observations about the mentee's progress in specific areas (Clark 2011). This may be wholly appropriate. However, it can often be more beneficial (in order to internalise the need to address a key area) to give the mentee the opportunity to reflect on their own progress. This can be done if the mentor simply asks them directly about which aspects of their teaching and learning they think they are performing best in, and having an open discussion about this.

Even more productive is the opportunity for a degree of critical reflexivity, where students can engage more fully with how they can fundamentally improve their performance in key areas. Differences in personality are a huge consideration at this stage. For instance, some mentees will find it difficult to accept praise, whereas others will not be very open to constructive criticism (Barnett 2011).

Reflection can be an invaluable tool when the mentor is not available to give immediate feedback and for particularly emotive aspects of the teaching and learning process. More introspective students can tend to turn every issue into a potential critical incident, while more extrovert students may trivialise potentially complex areas that would benefit from reflection.

Conclusion

Work-based learning is now the norm for the vast majority of postgraduate-level healthcare students. To get the most out of it, you need to focus your attention on:

- The overall process of education and how you as a student can address the learning outcomes of your particular postgraduate programme
- The professional relationships that drive the process of learning 'in situ' and how you engage and reflect on your experiential learning in practice
- The shaping of your own professionalism through learned experience and the recognition of your own strengths and weaknesses.

Fundamental to your experience will be your work with a mentor or clinical supervisor who can facilitate and direct your learning. In many instances, this learning process will shape the future direction of your employment.

5

Constructing a thesis or dissertation

Dr John Fulton

As part of a master's programme, students are expected to complete a project or a small-scale research study. The exact nature of this depends on the requirements of the particular course of study, and full details will be given in the course outline. However, this chapter will consider some very general principles that apply in most situations.

A key factor in successfully completing a thesis or dissertation is good time management. In my experience, mammoth last-minute sessions rarely work – when people think they can 'blitz it in a week!' or they leave writing up their dissertation until the week before the submission date. What *does* work is approaching your project in a systematic manner. Working on it regularly keeps it at the forefront of your mind and makes it more likely that you will plan your work systematically. For example, it is an excellent strategy to use a Gantt chart to plan when each section will be completed. It is also a good strategy to write while you are developing the study. Some sections of the final report (such as the literature review) can be written early on in the process. This strategy will both clarify your thinking and help your time management.

Structuring empirical studies

First we will consider empirical studies. These are studies that are 'based on, concerned with or verifiable by observation or experience rather than theory or pure logic' (*Oxford English Dictionary* 2014). In other words, they involve the collection of data. There are various types of data and of course the type of data will partly determine your approach to presenting your findings. However, while individual studies may be structured or presented in different ways, certain elements are always present and they are:

- An introduction in which you set out your aims
- A literature review in which you look at the work that has already been carried out or what is already known about the area of work

- An outline of your research approach – in other words, how your study will be structured or how you will go about answering your question
- Why you want or need to write about what you have found and present the results in a way that people can easily understand
- A discussion of the results, which means going back to your literature review to see if and how your work has added to existing knowledge.

Most reports follow this format, although these sections may not be easily discernible in all of them.

Introduction

In your introduction, you should state your idea and describe the general area you want to investigate. The introduction gives the broad outline and it is an opportunity to think about the background of the topic. For example, I carried out some research on boxing. The introduction gave me the opportunity to outline current thinking about boxing in the UK and the general state of the art. Your introduction also provides an opportunity to state where the idea for your research project has come from.

Literature review

For any project, you need a summary of the literature or what is known about the area you want to investigate. It is particularly important that you gather the most up-to-date and relevant information and ensure that it comes from reliable sources, based on original research (Aveyard 2010).

The following points are important regardless of how long the literature review is, but they are particularly important if the review is the entire study. You need to give some thought to the structure and focus of your literature review. It is not enough to read each paper and describe its findings. Rather, you need to organise it into themes and address them systematically. If you are doing one very large review, it may be that each chapter covers a particular theme.

It is also important to exercise a degree of critical judgement – that is, rather than simply describing the content of each paper, you should evaluate the quality of the work and the appropriateness or otherwise of the methodological approach. You need to summarise and identify gaps in your review. If you are going on to undertake your own research, the literature review is particularly important as it can help you shape and develop your own study.

It takes time and skill to unpick all this information, although there are some techniques that can make the job much easier. The Internet has greatly simplified this process but it can also overwhelm us with a lot of information. The only rule to follow is to 'work smarter', meaning that you need to take an efficient approach when gathering information.

Firstly, it is worth making friends with your subject librarian, as they will be able to point you in the correct direction and show you how to retrieve information in an efficient and effective manner. It is also useful to familiarise yourself with your university library's electronic material, as they will have databases that will link you with the key publications in the field. Secondly, familiarise yourself with the databases relating to your subject area. You should not be using Wikipedia or general sources on the Internet; you need to use specialist databases to access high-quality peer-reviewed journals.

When you put key words and terms into a database, they are used as the basis of the search and the information obtained is only as good as the terms. This is why it is good to use more than one term. For example, if you are looking for information on 'breast feeding', it might be useful to also try 'lactation', as some papers may use only one of these terms. Similarly, in teaching it might be useful to use 'teaching' and other terms such as 'pedagogy'. Although they are not really synonyms, they can still be used almost interchangeably so it might be helpful to use both. You can include 'and' or 'or' when combining key words; it is very useful to do more than one search and to play around with terms.

You also need to decide how far you are going back in your search, as many databases go back more than 50 years or so, and it would be impossible to look at all the information on a subject. You could limit yourself, say, to the past 10 years. In a rapidly developing field, this should give you an overview of all the up-to-date information. However, it does not mean that any information or papers published before that date are not of value. Some papers are seminal, meaning that they form the basis of much of the work done subsequently. Of course, if you know the subject area you will know the seminal works. Also, if a work is often quoted in the other papers you read, it is a good idea to seek it out, and read it and incorporate it in your review.

In addition, you will have to decide on the type of papers you are looking for and this will be partly determined by your area of study and the approaches people usually take in that field. For example, in medical research the randomised control trial is considered to be the gold standard. Other academic areas may value qualitative research, whereas in arts subjects philosophical enquiry may be highly respected. In healthcare, there is a clear hierarchy of evidence, with systematic reviews at the top (Petticrew & Roberts 2003). Although there is now a strong tradition of qualitative research in healthcare, medicine has not been a particularly strong supporter of qualitative research until fairly recently. However the tables are turning and the value of qualitative research is becoming increasingly recognised. It will be interesting to see where qualitative research is placed in subsequent revisions of this 'evidence hierarchy'.

The important point is that you should be able to recognise and identify the work that is most highly valued in your area of practice, and base your review on literature that is appropriate to your area of enquiry and your research questions. If you do this, you will be able to see the most up-to-date thinking in the area you are investigating.

You will of course have an idea of the area you want to study at the outset, and this will focus your literature review. Your review will also enable you to refine and focus your question or aims. You will be able to see which aspects of your subject have already been considered and which might need further exploration.

Research approaches

This section will consider the undertaking of research, especially research that involves people (or, to use the research term, 'human subjects'). This involves the type of information that will give you the answers to your questions or will address your particular focus. It is important to select an approach that is best suited to the area of enquiry. The two main types of approach are qualitative and quantitative.

Qualitative research involves looking in a fair amount of detail at a particular area or phenomenon. It is important that the situation is looked at in the real world (observed as it actually happens). To put it in another way, this type of research means looking holistically at an area of practice or a situation. It can also involve getting people to discuss their experiences or views of something in depth. This approach is useful if you wish to consider people's experiences and how the social world is negotiated (Fulton *et al.* 2013).

Quantitative research is, as the name suggests, an attempt to quantify or count something. Rather than examining the situation holistically, a particular aspect is considered in some detail. It can be used to determine trends and patterns or the relationship between two parts or, to use the research term, two variables. This means that the situation is broken down into its component parts. Each of these parts is compared with the other, or the relationship between the two may be examined (Fulton *et al.* 2013).

Both these types of research suggest going to talk to people or observing them or in some way interacting with them as a way of obtaining information. It is of course also possible to get information from documentary sources or from analysis of newspaper or magazine articles. Plowright (2012) puts this very succinctly and provides a table in which he outlines the different type of research information that can be obtained. Plowright also states that to gain information one asks questions, or observes something or looks at artefacts. Rather than discuss qualitative and quantitative approaches, he differentiates them as 'structured' (quantitative) and 'unstructured' (qualitative) approaches. From the standpoint, the degree of structure you require for your investigation will determine whether you take a qualitative or quantitative approach.

It is becoming increasingly common to mix the two approaches (qualitative and quantitative) in one study, each approach providing information that addresses the research question in a different way. This can be extremely helpful. For example, many researchers carry out a qualitative piece of research to find out the main issues and, on this basis, go on to develop a questionnaire in order to get quantitative date. However, before getting too enthusiastic about this idea, you need to remember the constraints of your course and the time you have available. Bearing these factors in mind, it is often best to keep things fairly straightforward and stick to either a qualitative or quantitative approach.

To give an example, I was interested in boxing as an activity and in particular on why people took up the sport and how it could interact with other areas of young men's lives. (When I did the study it was almost exclusively a male sport, and today there are many more female boxers.) I found there was very little literature about the subject. To investigate, I therefore needed to explore the situation holistically, which led to a qualitative piece of research (Fulton 2011). I could have compiled a questionnaire and distributed it to the various boxing clubs in the area and determined the various patterns (such as representation of age ranges, types of occupations, the particular social class of many of the informants, and other information about numbers of bouts). The type of information I could obtain would differ, depending on the approach, but both could be equally valuable. Of course, I also could look at documentation and information collected by the Amateur and Professional Boxing Association. What is important is that some thought is given to the method of collecting data and the type of information you want, and that you collect this is in a systematic way.

Master's students often rush out and collect data, and then find themselves surrounded by a great deal of information and don't have a clue what to do with it! This is why it is important to plan ahead and think about the data you will need, how you will collect it and how you will analyse it. In qualitative studies, the data is usually analysed as the research process unfolds and the analysis will shape the collection of the subsequent data. In a quantitative study, you might be using a questionnaire, for example, and distributing it to large numbers of people. You won't have the luxury of altering it after the event, if you later realise that some questions are ambiguous or have been misinterpreted. It is important to pilot the questionnaire first and sort out these issues before sending out the main questionnaire. It is also very important to think of what you want to get out the questionnaires. Broadly (as stated previously), you might be looking for general patterns or trends or you might be looking for relationships between variables. All these aspects will help determine the types of questions you will ask. Planning is therefore very important and time spent in planning can reap many rewards.

You also need to remember that while your research is extremely important to you, it does not have the same priority for everyone else! This includes the people who are going to give you the information you want. Theoretically, questionnaires can provide a lot of information very quickly but in reality there is often a low response rate. Similarly, with qualitative interviews, people may agree at first but it is not a priority for them, and they will quickly cancel if they get a better offer or if something else crops up. It is worth bearing this in mind and allowing for this in your planning and scheduling.

The sample (meaning those who will answer your questions or who you are going to observe) is very important. You will not be able to ask questions of everyone who is involved – for example, all the people who have asthma or all premier league footballers. You will therefore need to select a sample that represents a particular group. You need to think about the type and purpose of your sample. Broadly speaking, in quantitative research, you are seeking a representative sample. In qualitative research, you are looking for people who can give you certain types of information, sometimes called a purposeful sample (Neuman 2002).

Often in research we are interested in what are called 'vulnerable groups', such as people of a particular age range or people who have a particular condition. Ethical approval is required before carrying out research in order to show that any ethical issues have been duly considered. Your university will have an ethics committee and clear guidelines on ethical issues. You will need to show you that have considered these issues and, most importantly, that your respondents will come to no harm from participating in the research.

In addition, if you want to access specific groups of people you will also need ethical approval from particular agencies. For example, if you are looking at schoolchildren then you need approval from their schools and the relevant education authority. For patients or if you are exploring a health-related issue, you will need to approach the NHS ethics committee. You cannot do your research without this approval and it can take some time to get it. You therefore need to build this into your plans and, at worst, it can sometimes mean not accessing a particular sample of people. Often, if formal ethical approval is not needed, people assume that there are no ethical issues involved at all and of course this not the case. Regardless of whether or not formal ethical approval is needed, you have to show that you are concerned about ethical issues and have considered them in the design of the study.

Your research approach will be the subject of a chapter in your final report. In this chapter, you will need to outline all the above issues and demonstrate how they have been considered.

Presenting your results

Having collected the raw data, you will have to analyse it. As stated earlier, you should plan the analysis from the beginning, as it is easy to be overwhelmed by large amounts of data. If you are using statistics, Statistical Package for the Social Sciences (SPSS) is available at most universities. If the data is inputted in the correct format, it can be analysed within seconds of pushing a button. But you need to know how to input the data and what tests to select, and this is where you will need training and help.

Qualitative data can be vast and cumbersome and its analysis does require training, but it becomes much more manageable if you analyse it as you go along. There are several computer packages that can help with this. Different qualitative approaches can indicate the ways in which the analysis can be carried out, but the basis of qualitative data is the establishment and development of themes. The way these themes are analysed and combined can be complex but achievable and very interesting, and some training is required.

The second challenge is presenting the results in a way that is understandable and accessible to the reader. Different techniques are required for qualitative and quantitative approaches. Quantitative results tend to be presented in the form of tables and charts. They are also 'stand-alone' so no explanation is necessarily provided. The results and their trends need to be very clear. Statistical packages will enable you to produce graphs and charts but the reader needs to be able to understand them. You will therefore have to decide whether or not to include only summary tables, and how much or how little supporting information needs to be provided. It may also be that you provide a summary at the end of the results to highlight the trends and what relationships, if any, have been established. There are many guides to SPSS (for example, UCLA 2014) but make sure the guide you consult addresses the version of SPSS you are using – a mistake I once made!

Qualitative data requires a slightly different strategy. In qualitative research, a number of themes are established, all of which are named. There are many textbooks that outline approaches to analysing qualitative data – for example, Huberman and Miles (2002). The meaning of the theme or name is not always immediately apparent (for instance, sometimes a common everyday word is used slightly differently). You also need evidence, either from quotes from an interview or observational notes. Novice researchers often think it is enough to give a heading and some quotes. However, this is unfortunately not enough and a level of explanation is also required. It is important not to use too many quotes from your research. Use enough to provide supporting evidence but do not fill pages with quotes; it is better to weave them into your explanation.

Whether your approach is qualitative or quantitative, the reader must have a good idea of your findings. This will lead them onto your penultimate chapter, the discussion.

Discussion and conclusion

This is the point where people tend to run out of steam and think 'I have said it all already'! However, the discussion is extremely important, as this where you are indicating the value of your work. What you need to do is to return to the literature and re-evaluate it in the light of your findings. (This is another reason why you should undertake a good literature review at the outset.) The more familiar you are with the literature, the better placed you are to assess your work it. In this discussion section you need to be evaluative and clear about your claims. Whether you are producing a systematic review or a research study, it is important to discuss what you have found out in the course of the investigation.

This is also the place to mention the limitations of your work – and there will always be limitations. By definition, you will have undertaken a relatively small study and your resources are limited so it is important to acknowledge this. As I was once advised, 'Someone will always point out the limitations so you may as well get in first!'

The conclusion is usually a separate chapter and this is where you will summarise you work, your findings and the conclusions you have reached. Recommendations are often included. For instance, if you have explored a practice area, you may wish to include practice-based recommendations and suggestions as to how your study could be developed.

Another huge issue is referencing. Any academic piece of work needs to be well and accurately referenced, which is easier said than done. There are now various reference management tools available, such as Endnote and Zotero, which make the task considerably easier. You will need training in these but the time investment is well worth it, as they can simplify matter considerably. If you don't use referencing management software, do be meticulous in recording your references. If you don't record them as you go, it will be difficult if not impossible to find them in retrospect (and I say this from experience!).

Now, having completed the research and the writing of the report, you are entitled to a well-deserved rest but only for a few days! Before submission, you need to read through your work, remove typographical errors, delete any repetition, improve any wording that is unclear and so on. This can make a huge difference to your work. Only when the final version is handed in can you relax.

Systematic reviews

So far, we have only considered empirical studies – that is, studies based on observation or, more specifically, the collection of data. We will now examine projects that involve the use of secondary sources or previously published studies. This type of investigation is called a systematic review. It is similar to a literature review but it is carried out in a much more rigorous and systematic way. There is a website called PRISMA, which stands for 'Preferred Reporting Items for Systematic Reviews and Meta-Analyses'. PRISMA contains much useful information on different types of systematic review and how to conduct one (PRISMA 2009). It's best to think of a systematic review as a research study but one that is carried out using papers, rather than people, as the object of investigation. To undertake a systematic review, the researcher needs to establish a question or a very clear focus for the investigation. The literature review should be established, and the research question refined in the light of it.

Having established the research question, with possible sub-question, the next step is to identify the papers and research studies that you are going to investigate. As with a literature review, you will need to be clear about your inclusion and exclusion criteria, both in terms of the area of investigation and the methodological approach. It is common to undertake the review based on one methodology – for instance, using only systematic reviews or only randomised control trials. This will depend on the question and is another reason why the question should be very focused. The literature needs to be searched and then you can apply your inclusion/exclusion criteria. The papers have to be screened and those not addressing the exact question, or not using the particular methodological approach, should be excluded. Typically this can take the number of papers from over 100 to about 25. The remaining papers are assessed for their methodological quality. The assessment for quality is done against pre-set criteria, and those not meeting the standard are excluded. This narrows the number even further, and means that only the very best evidence is considered.

Each paper is considered in some detail and the particular results are outlined, trends are very clearly demonstrated and the overall pattern is thus established. The next step is that the results are analysed as one. This process differs, depending on whether it is a qualitative or quantitative study. When undertaking a statistical analysis, a 'meta-analysis' is carried out. This means that the statistics from all the studies are combined and analysed together, and the overall pattern or trend is identified (Hemingway 2009). This type of research can be very powerful and offers a good way of dealing with papers that have conflicting findings. Systematic reviews and meta-analysis are becoming increasingly common in many disciplines, but the approach was pioneered in medicine. The Internet-based Cochrane Library contains many of these systematic reviews. The Cochrane Library is a source that is well worth checking out, as it has numerous examples of systematic reviews (Cochrane 2014).

Less well established but becoming increasingly popular is the systematic review of qualitative studies (Sandelowski *et al.* 1997). In doing such a review, the principles outlined in the preceding paragraph are followed. However, as statistics are not being used, a meta-analysis cannot really be undertaken. Instead, a 'meta-synthesis' is carried out. Qualitative studies tend to identify themes or patterns. In a meta-synthesis, the themes or patterns from the selected studies are combined and expanded. Again, the central question and the quality of the papers are very important, as you should end up with a very powerful summary of several papers and trends being clearly identified.

One drawback of systematic reviews is what is called 'publication bias'. This means that there is a tendency to publish positive results; and if something is shown not to work, it is less likely to be published. For example, if there are 100 studies on a question and 20 show positive findings and 80 show negative results, more positive ones may still be published. People undertaking systematic reviews are very aware of this and look for unpublished work in order to determine the real trends. The constraints of your project might not allow for this but it is something you need to be aware of as an issue and acknowledge it as a possible limitation.

Managing your supervisor

You will be given a supervisor to support and help you in your work. Your supervisor is a valuable resource and it is important that you use this resource to your full advantage. To do this, you need to meet regularly with your supervisor and it is your responsibility to ensure that this happens. Your supervisor will be interested in your project but it will not be their main priority. They will be extremely busy with other things. You should therefore find out the best time to see them and make regular appointments. Try not to turn up without an appointment, as you will inevitably find them busy and distracted.

You also need to use appointments to their full advantage by coming prepared with questions and areas you wish to explore. If you have written something and want your supervisor to comment on it, send it in a few days before your meeting. This will give them time to read it and comment. Don't send something to your supervisor at midnight and expect comments for your 9am meeting! Importantly, if you are unsure about anything, do contact your supervisor. A quick email exchange can often save you hours of work and worry.

Most universities allocate certain hours for supervision and you need to manage this time. You might want regular meetings when you are planning your work, perhaps each week, and then less regular meetings when you are collecting data, and then more frequently when you are completing the study. Again, individual universities will have rules about the number of drafts the supervisor will comment on. However, most will allow the supervisor to comment on a draft of each chapter, and see and comment on the final version. This is another reason to approach the writing systematically and not to leave it all to the last minute, to allow time for your supervisor to read and comment on your work.

Conclusion

To summarise:

- Plan your time and work regularly and often
- Take note of your ideas and where they came from
- Familiarise yourself with the available literature
- On the basis of your literature review, refine your research question or aims
- Choose a methodology that will best address your research question or aims
- Determine the skills you need, look for any gaps and get the approprite training
- Spend time on your report and remember that someone has to read it so you should make it interesting and intelligible
- Use critical judgement about your own work
- Manage your supervisor
- Don't leave it all until the last minute!

6

Disseminating academic work

Dr Judith Kuit

There are many reasons, both intrinsic and extrinsic, to disseminate your research. From a personal point of view, it is very satisfying to see your name in print and it provides an acknowledgement by your peers that your work is worthwhile and you have been accepted in the world of research and scholarship.

The first time you submit your work for publication or presentation, you will feel very apprehensive but you should see it as an opportunity to receive feedback on your work from a much wider audience than you would normally encounter. Although this feedback will be critical, it will also be constructive. You need to be able to take this criticism in the spirit in which it is offered and accept that it isn't personal, even though it may sometimes feel as if it is. It is highly unlikely that any journal or conference would accept submitted work without some element of criticism because that is what academic colleagues do for a living. Remember that the main benefit of your university education is to gain the ability to construct an objective argument and to critically evaluate text.

The benefits of disseminating your work

The central purpose of your research and/or your thesis is to propose something that is new and open for critical discussion, and this is what you do when you disseminate your work. At postgraduate level, your research should challenge the status quo. Critical evaluation of the work (by yourself and others) is part of the process of improving and developing what you have done. Your research is built upon the work of others and you demonstrate how sound your research is through critical discussion of your findings in the context of other academic literature. If others had never published their work, you would have nothing with which to compare your findings. In this situation, how would research develop and progress? You need to publish your work because if you don't disseminate it to your peers then there is no point in undertaking it in the first place. If you keep research hidden, it cannot be validated by others and it becomes fruitless.

If your work has been published and critically reviewed and accepted by your peers, you will be in a much stronger position by the time you go to your viva (oral examination on your thesis). You will have rehearsed the arguments and defended your thesis already. If your work has previously been accepted as worthy of publication, you are less likely to fail a viva or have to carry out extensive rewrites of your work – because it has been deemed worthy of publication beforehand.

Another advantage of disseminating your work is that it encourages you to practise writing in an academic style. Most postgraduate students are very anxious about writing up their dissertation or thesis, and may delay this task because it is such a big undertaking. But if you are disseminating your work for a conference or a paper, the amount of writing will be smaller and more focused and you will have to meet the deadline of the publication. All these intrinsic factors will encourage you to start writing, and will also help you approach the writing up of your thesis in a structured, planned way.

There are other extrinsic factors that will also stimulate your motivation. The strongest of these is your need to gain employment, once you graduate. You need to actively build up and strengthen your CV and network (Vitae 2013), and disseminating your work will help you do this. This will also be invaluable for raising your personal profile and marketing yourself so that you can get a job.

Starting small and local

Your first attempt at dissemination doesn't necessarily have to involve publishing a full research paper or presenting at a national or international conference. You should start small in order to build your confidence and develop your presentation skills. Many universities host research student conferences to give their students an opportunity to practise presenting and discussing their work. These tend to cover a wide area of research, which may not be specifically relevant to your work but will still enable you to practise your presentation skills and describe your work.

Most universities have departmental seminars, which are usually non-threatening, low-profile informal events, sometimes held over lunch, where researchers can present their work. You should volunteer to present at one of these, either in your own department or in another, to practise presenting to an audience and discussing and getting feedback on your work from others who are interested in a similar field.

Submitting work to a conference

Once you feel sufficiently confident about the quality of your research and your ability to withstand public scrutiny, you can consider submitting your work to a conference. You should get advice from your research supervisor and choose which conference would be most appropriate for you and which part of your work to submit. If you are accepted, many conferences give you the pre-option of presenting a poster or an oral presentation. However, some conferences only tell you after you have been selected which type of presentation you have been offered. If you have a choice, the option you select will depend on your level of confidence. If you feel confident about giving an oral presentation in front of an audience, select that route. If you don't, then present a poster, but you shouldn't assume that a poster presentation is second best. You may get fewer people coming to look at your poster but those who do are likely to be more interested in your work specifically and may wish to discuss your findings one-to-one. If your conference abstract has been accepted, you will need to prepare carefully for the event.

Giving an oral presentation at a conference

If you are giving an oral presentation, practise it frequently in front of your colleagues beforehand. You need to ensure that your presentation is structured and has a clear beginning, middle and end. Imagine that you are telling a story but the story is your research and you are telling it to a knowledgeable audience. Start by saying who you are, and clearly state the aim of your research and its purpose, thus answering the why question. Then explain how you did the research, what you found and why it is relevant.

You may only have ten minutes for your presentation so you need to be clear and succinct in order to make a good impression. Your slides need to be readable from a distance so you should use a sans serif font, black text on a white background or blue text on a cream background. Don't use distracting visuals or lurid colours. It detracts from your work and looks amateurish, which is not the impression you wish to create. Try to submit a copy of your presentation to the conference beforehand so that it can be copied and given out to the audience before you start. Remember to include all your contact details on this so that listeners can contact you afterwards.

When you give your talk, you should look at your audience and speak clearly so that everyone can hear you. You may feel nervous but if you speak too quietly and too quickly, the audience will struggle to hear what is being said. Try to memorise your talk but take your notes with you to the podium in case your mind goes blank. The clear message to your audience should be that your research is interesting and relevant so do your best to look enthusiastic and motivated as you present. If you look dull and bored by your work, others will feel the same, so try to smile and look positive. You may feel too nervous or embarrassed to look at your audience and it can be very off-putting if someone in the audience is not paying attention. To avoid these problems, just focus on a mid-point on the wall at the back of the room and you will appear to be looking at someone.

At the end of the presentation, there will be an opportunity for audience members to ask a couple of questions and it can be nerve-racking if you don't know the answers. This is another reason why it is a good idea to practise your talk in front of critical colleagues beforehand. If you are genuinely stuck for an answer, just turn the question back on the questioner. Say that they have raised an interesting point which you hadn't considered and ask if they have a view on it themselves.

After your presentation, make a point of talking to the person who asked you the most interesting questions and continue the discussion of your work if there is time. Think of it as dropping a pebble in a pond and seeing where the ripples will go. You don't know where this will lead in terms of your future career development, as this person will probably remember you and your research. If nothing else, you will have started to develop a network of people who are interested in your work. The more specialised your research, the fewer people are likely to work in it. Therefore the more people you can make contact and network with, the more likely you are to come across someone who may know about other research opportunities or job vacancies in your subject area.

Giving a poster presentation at a conference

If you are presenting a poster, then (like an oral presentation) it should have a clear structure with a definite beginning, middle and end. It should be easy to read quickly and have an obvious flow or sequence of information. A poster is not an advertisement, it is a mini-research paper, so don't use garish colours that make it difficult to read. It should be readable from two metres away so font size and colour are important. The conference organisers will give you specifications about the overall size of the poster.

You could use a provocative statement or an interesting and/or relevant photograph or diagram to attract people's attention. This is particularly important at a large conference, where hundreds of posters may be displayed. Most readers will probably only spend five to ten minutes looking at your poster so you need to have a high impact factor. You could also bring A4 print-outs of your poster or a summary of your work, with clear contact details, to use as a hand-out.

Although presenting a poster might seem less nerve-racking than giving an oral presentation, it will require you to be friendly and to start conversations with readers who are likely to be complete strangers. You will need to make them relax around your poster and you can't afford to miss any opportunities to network with future potential employers or colleagues. A good opening line is 'Would you like me to talk through the findings with you?' or 'Is this an area that is of particular interest to you?' A question like this should help to break the ice and lead into a more natural conversation. It might not lead anywhere but at least it will increase the chances of them remembering you.

Actively attending a conference

Don't take a passive approach to conferences. You should do far more than simply give a presentation and listen to other people giving their presentations. You need to be much more active, as this is a unique opportunity to network and to raise your profile. Planning is very important and this should start early on. Well before the conference takes place, think about what you want to get out of it, in addition to listing your presentation on your CV (Gannon-Leary & Smailes 2009).

You may want the opportunity to network and meet potential future employers, colleagues or collaborators. There may be someone at the conference who could be your future external examiner at your viva and it could be useful to see what sort of person they are and whether you fee comfortable with them. In order to find this out, you need to check the delegate list, which is usually given out at the registration desk on the first day. The key speakers at the conference will be mentioned on the conference website well beforehand and you will easily be able to check them out on the Internet to see if any of them are in your particular field.

When you have identified the people you would like to talk to, think of questions that you would like to ask them and/or contact them before the conference and ask if you can discuss your work with them. Remember to take a business card or an abstract of your research with you. Again, this should include your contact details so that you can give it to them and this will help them to remember you. If this one-to-one approach feels too pushy for you, then read through the conference abstracts, working out which ones will be the most relevant and useful for you to attend and plan out your schedule. Once you have worked out which people you would like to see, think of some questions that you could ask them at the session. Many conferences now have a blog that is open before the conference so you can contact people before the event starts. It is useful to continue with this during the conference so remember to take your laptop with you and make notes as you go.

While you are at the conference, make sure that you have your name badge on at all times so that other delegates can see who you are. Go to the informal social areas so you can start talking to other attendees and making contacts. You could ask other people if they have travelled far or if this is their first time in the venue. These useful icebreaker questions can easily start conversations that soon lead on to more interesting topics.

Conferences are deliberately organised with gaps in the schedule so that delegates can socialise and network. Make the most of these opportunities and remember to be positive and enthusiastic. You may find that you had a question planned to ask at a session but there wasn't enough time for you to ask it or you were too nervous to try. If this is the case, try to approach the presenter in a more informal setting, saying that you found the presentation very interesting and that you wanted to ask, etc. If there are plans for informal socialising after the conference or a conference dinner, go along so that you can meet people in relaxing surroundings. Attending the plenary session at a conference gives you a shared topic to start discussions with others and this can be followed up if the discussion proves fruitful.

When you leave the conference, make sure that you contact the people who you wish to maintain links with. It is useful to keep a note of each person's contact details and the reasons why you may wish to contact them again, either immediately or in the future. Each conference is an ideal networking opportunity so make the most of it. You will find that it is as much who you know as what you know that helps you to achieve success. The Vitae website (2013) has some very valuable information on raising your profile in this way.

Publishing in a journal

Having disseminated your work at a conference, the next step is to publish your research in a peer-reviewed academic journal. Publishing your work isn't just about dissemination. It is also expected by your supervisor, department and any future employer that your work should be of a sufficiently high standard to withstand critical evaluation. It is even a requirement in some countries, where a PhD cannot be awarded unless the work has been previously published (Smith 2012).

Realistically, you therefore have little choice but to publish if you wish to develop your career, and this should stimulate your intrinsic motivation to do so. Publishing in an academic journal may seem like a big step, but if your work has been included in a conference then it will have already had some form of peer review. You can therefore predict that others will also find it interesting and worthy of publication. It is accepted academic practice to present your work in progress at a conference and, when the work is complete, you submit it for publication in an academic journal.

Which journal to select?

This may seem like an odd step to take initially but inexperienced authors often write a paper, then send it around to various journals to see if they will publish it, and then wonder why it has been rejected by everyone. The first step is to select the most appropriate journal for your research. The choice could be obvious – if most of the research in your subject area is published in one journal. If it isn't obvious, then you need to select the journal that will have the greatest impact in terms of reader profile (Smith 2012). This means that you have to read many journals to identify which one is most appropriate for the topic. Your supervisor should be able to help you make this choice because if you do submit a paper to the wrong type of journal it will be returned to you very quickly by the editor and you will have wasted your time as well as theirs.

Nowadays you can usually choose whether to submit to a paper-based journal and/or an online publication. Clearly, submitting something online has the potential to lead to a quicker publication and a wider dissemination of your work but that is not always an advantage. McDonald (2011) suggests that disseminating online is more likely to lead to others progressing your ideas before you do, or plagiarising the work you have done. This can be a real problem if your thesis is published online and someone else copies it and tries to submit it as their own. Universities find it very difficult to prevent this.

Turning your coursework into a publication

Hall (2007) has some very sound advice about turning your coursework into journal articles. Whilst there are many similarities between writing coursework and writing a journal article, there are also some fundamental differences. Firstly, coursework tends to be written in a defensive manner, clearly articulating the argument, using the references cited. This is because you are defending your work against an examiner. In contrast, a journal article will still include references but will relate them more to the findings in the discussion. Consequently, a journal article is shorter and more pithy. Secondly, coursework is writer-centric. It is partly about you learning how to write and demonstrating how you do this to your supervisors and examiners. Meanwhile, the main purpose of writing a journal article is that someone will want to read it, which is why the topic is so important. Journals wouldn't get many readers if the topics were so irrelevant that no one wanted to read any of them. Once you have considered both these points, you can begin the writing process.

Academic writing

It is taken as a given that your writing must be grammatically correct, with good use of punctuation and spelling. If it isn't and/or you are writing in a foreign or second language, you should seek help. Most universities offer support to students who are struggling to develop their language skills and their ability to write so make sure you take advantage of any help that is available.

Academic writing is a specific skill that you need to acquire very quickly (if you don't already have it from your undergraduate degree), as it is accepted practice that you will use it in your thesis and to publish. It is customary to write academic text in the third person, using the passive voice and the past tense.

Having said that, some (Hartley 2008, p.4) would argue that:

Academic writing is:
- *unnecessarily complicated*
- *pompous, long-winded, technical*
- *impersonal, authoritative, humourless*
- *elitist, and excludes outsiders.*

But it can be:
- *appropriate in specific circumstances*
- *easier for non-native speakers to follow.*

It is certainly true that in some subject areas (such as education and the arts and humanities) using the first person is an acceptable practice, particularly if reflective writing is required. But in technology, science and engineering, writing in the third person, past tense, passive voice is mandatory. Whatever your viewpoint, academic writing is a skill you must develop in order to disseminate your work. The more academic texts and journals you read, the more familiar you will become with academic writing. This is possibly because as you read, you hear the words in your head, and the writing style becomes familiar and embedded.

Most academic writing is a combination of three different styles (Murphy 2010):

- Narrative writing that describes a subject
- Exposition or informative writing that explains, analyses or interprets
- Persuasive writing, which you present and develop your point of view.

Having previously submitted assignments, you will have become practised in these forms and this will help you to develop your work for publication.

You must learn to construct an argument in your academic writing, providing objective evidence for and against the point that you are trying to make so that your research claims can be evaluated in the context of the literature. If you make claims that are unsupported by any evidence and merely anecdotal, it is unlikely that anyone will accept your work. Your arguments should be coherent and well structured so that your work is logical to read. This means that you need to be able to effectively summarise and paraphrase the key points of the literature that you have read in order to construct a scholarly argument.

The writing needs a logical and coherent structure, with a clear beginning, middle and end, with cohesion so that one paragraph naturally flows into the next. Reading your writing out aloud will help you with this.

The way you approach the actual act of writing is up to you. Some people prefer to write by hand and then type it up on the computer. Others prefer to write straight on to the screen. If you can do this, it will save you a lot of time in the long run. When you first start writing, it might seem like an insurmountable task, and you may try to avoid it at all costs.

Some people are divergent thinkers and like to grow their writing by starting with one point and developing it organically from there. Others are convergent thinkers and prefer to structure the work and use the outline as a framework to support the writing. The secret is to start small and do a little every day. You don't have to start at the beginning and work your way through to the end. Try starting at a point that doesn't require too much intellectual effort, such as a narrative section describing a method. If you write a little every day, it becomes a less onerous task. It also keeps the subject fresh in your mind so that you can easily sit down and start writing again, instead of trying to remember at which point you ended. When you finish writing for the day, you may find it helpful to leave a few words at the end, as clues to what you want to say next.

This chapter has only given a very brief summary of how to undertake academic writing. If you want further guidance, there are many helpful texts available on the subject (Hartley 2008, Murray 2009, Murphy 2010, Soles 2010).

How to write an article for a journal

When you have selected the journal, you need to obtain the journal's instructions for contributors as they will provide specific information about length, style, format etc. and you must write and submit the paper using these style guidelines (Good, 2013). You should write a first draft of the paper and give it to a colleague or your supervisor for informal peer-review and revise the paper in light of this feedback. The article itself should be written in a similar way to your thesis:

1. Abstract: summary of the research

2. Key words: vital words to aid selection by readers when doing searches

3. Introduction: providing a context and a clear aim

4. Review of the literature: this should be current and relevant

5. Methodology: description and justification of the process

6. Limitations of the research: showing scope and scale of the research

7. Findings: including diagrams, figures or tables if appropriate

8. Discussion: the significance of the findings and conclusions

9. References: current and in the requested format

If the writing of a full paper seems to be an insurmountable task then break it down into sections and write a little every day until you complete the paper. You don't necessarily have to write it in the order given above, start with what you feel most comfortable with and build it up in sections but always end with the abstract as this must be written succinctly and accurately to attract readers.

Hartley, (2008), Murray (2009) and Murphy (2010), all provide extensive guidance on writing a journal article and writing for publication.

Submitting an article to a journal

When you and your supervisor are both satisfied with your article, submit it to the journal that you have selected along with a covering letter. Don't think that you will save time by sending the article to more than one journal at the same time. Editors communicate with each other and if editors find out your article is also under consideration by another journal, they will reject it out of hand (Smith 2012). Wait until one journal rejects it before sending it to another one.

If an editor thinks your paper has the potential to be published, it will be circulated to reviewers to evaluate. Journal editors normally use a blind review system in which the reviewers do not know the identity of the writers and vice versa. This process can take a number of weeks so don't panic if you don't hear anything for a while, and don't expect the feedback to say that it is perfect and doesn't require any changes. Reviewers quite often give contradictory advice and it is likely that all reviewers and the editor will be highly critical of your work. As stated at the beginning of this chapter, you shouldn't take this criticism personally; it is intended to be constructive. Respond to the criticisms in a positive way. Rewrite as required and re-submit the article. If you have addressed their criticisms, it is highly likely to be accepted at this point. Then all you have to do is wait for the publication to come out. Many journals have a set number of issues per year and it may take several months for your article to appear in print but if it is accepted, you can still include it in your CV saying 'in press' where the year would normally go.

Converting your thesis into a book

In the humanities and social sciences, it is more common to convert your thesis into a book, rather than write two or three journal articles, but that doesn't mean that the process is any easier. As Haslam (2013a, 2013b, 2013c) points out, an examiner has to read your thesis but it is unlikely that someone would pay for the privilege of doing so. A publisher is more likely to publish a book that is based on your thesis, as this is more likely to be popular with readers. As you would with a journal, select a publisher who is more likely to publish books in your subject area and write to a named editor with an outline of your proposal, the intended market and what makes it different from other texts in the field. The process is similar to that of submitting an article, in that peer review is involved and feedback will have to be addressed. The whole process will take several months to complete but to see a book with your name on the cover on your bookshelf or coffee table is very satisfying and it will obviously make the ideal Christmas gift for relatives and friends!

Writing a review

You may be reading this chapter and appreciating the value of dissemination but your research isn't ready to disseminate yet, so what can you do to raise your profile and practise your writing skills? One option is to offer to write a review article on your research topic. Having read around the subject and carried out a literature review, you should be very knowledgeable on this topic. Even if you haven't done any writing on your thesis at this stage, focusing on writing a review for others will help you to write your own literature review when necessary.

Start by contacting the editor of the journal that is most relevant to your work and offer a topic for review or perhaps a few topics in a general area. The worst that can happen is that the editor will say 'no' so you have little to lose. Even if you get a rejection, perhaps the editor will remember you and come back to you later and ask you to review something for the journal. If you feel that providing a review article is too big a step at this point, you could offer to review a new book instead. Most journals will have a reviews editor who will receive many unsolicited newly published books and who will be looking for someone to review a text who is knowledgeable about the subject matter. Not only will this help you to develop your academic writing skills; providing a well-balanced, constructive, non-personal critical evaluation of the work will also enable you to develop your own ability to critically reflect. You may also get a free book!

Public engagement

Increasingly, universities or sponsors of your work request that you engage with the public in disseminating your work. This may be for political reasons, particularly if you work for a public sector organisation or in an area that is highly topical or controversial. Alternatively, you may just wish to talk about what you are doing and disseminate your work in a less formal way. This could be in a non-specialist magazine, by going into schools, working with clubs or patient groups, or presenting at exhibitions or festivals. Whatever the venue, it is a good idea to take the opportunity to explain in a straightforward way what it is you do in your work. Thinking of imaginative ways in which you can explain this to others, who are non-specialists, will improve your own understanding of the topic. The Vitae website (2013) offers many useful suggestions about engaging with the public.

Conclusion

This chapter discusses many reasons for disseminating your work and most of them are personal. Those that aren't personal tend not to be reasons but requirements! So, wherever the pressures come from, you should take every opportunity to disseminate your work.

References

Ainley, P. & Rainbird, H. (eds) (2014). *Apprenticeship: Towards a New Paradigm of Learning.* Abingdon: Routledge.

Alinier, G, Harwood, C., Harwood, P., Montague, S., Huish, E., Ruparelia, K., & Antuofermo, M. (2014). Immersive clinical simulation inundergraduate health care interprofessional education: Knowledge and perceptions. *Clinical Simulation in Nursing.* **10** (4), 205–216.

Armstrong, C. (2007). Getting your academic work published. http://www.jobs.ac.uk/careers-advice/working-in-higher-education/640/getting-your-academic-work-published/ (Accessed 31 October 2013).

Aveyard, H. (2010). *Doing a literature reviewin health and social care: A practical guide.* Maidenhead: McGraw-Hill International.

Barlow, J. & Fleischer, S. (2011). Student absenteeism: whose responsibility? *Innovations in Education and Teaching International.* **48** (3), 227–37.

Barnett, N. (2011). Learning and development-resources-mentoring. *Pharmaceutical Journal.* **286** (7641), 202

Becker, L. (2004). *How to Manage your Postgraduate Course.* Palgrave Study Guides. Basingstoke: Palgrave Macmillan.

Birenbaum, M. & Amdur, L. (1999). Reflective active learning in a graduate course on assessment. *Higher Education Research and Development.* **18** (2), 201–18.

Bowling, A. (2009). *Research Methods in Health: Investigating Health and Health Services.* Maidenhead: McGraw-Hill International.

Bulut, H., Hisar, F. & Demir, S.G. (2010). Evaluation of mentorship programme in nursing education: A pilot study in Turkey. *Nurse Education Today.* **30** (8), 756–62.

Chou, C.L., Hirschmann, K., Fortin, A.H. & Lichstein, P.R. (Jul 2014). The impact of a faculty learning community on professional and personal development: the facilitator training program of the American Academy on Communication in Healthcare. *Academic Medicine.* **89** (7), 1051–56.

Clark, R.A.F. (2011). Teacher, supervisor, adviser, or mentor quest. *Journal of Investigative Dermatology.* **131** (9), 1779–80.

Cochrane (2014). The Cochrane Collaboration. http://www.cochrane.org/ (Accessed 30 June 2014).

Daycare Trust (2013). Last update, Parent Information. http://www.daycaretrust.org.uk/pages/parent-information.html (Accessed 10 January 2013).

De Bono, E. (1999). *Six Thinking Hats.* London, Penguin.

De Bono, E. & Zimbalist, E. (2010). *Lateral Thinking.* London: Viking.

Department for Business, Innovation and Skills (BIS) (2011). White Paper: Higher Education: Students at the Heart of the System. London: The Stationery Office.

Dunbar-Morris, Dr H. (2010). *Managing Students' Expectations of University.* 1994 Group, Student Experience Policy Group. London: Jisc.

ECCTIS (2013). Diagram of higher education qualification levels in England, Wales and Northern Ireland. http://www.ecctis.co.uk/europass/documents/ds_chart.pdf (Accessed 10 January 2013).

Ellis, A.K. (2014). *Research on Educational Innovations.* Abingdon: Routledge.

ESIB (2003). ESIB and the Bologna Process – Creating a European Higher Education Area for and with Students. Berlin, 18–19 September 2003. In *Realising the European Higher Education Area.* Conference of European Ministers Responsible for Higher Education. Documentation. Bielefeld: W. Bertelsmann Verlag. 72–83

Eunjung, O. & Reeves, T.C. (2014). Generational differences and the integration of technology in learning, instruction, and performance. *Handbook of Research on Educational Communications and Technology.* New York: Springer. 819–28.

Fallon, H. & Breen, E. (2013). Academic publishing: Maximising library expertise,resources and services. *AISHE-J.* **5** (1), 1131–39.

Fulton, J. (2011). What's your worth? The development of capital in british boxing. *European Journal for Sport and Society.* **8** (3), 193–218.

Fulton J., Kuit J., Sanders G. & Smith P. (2012). The role of the Professional Doctorate in developing professional practice. *Journal of Nursing Management.* **20**, 130–39

Fulton, J., Kuit, J., Sanders, G. & Smith, P. (2013). *The Professional Doctorate: A Practical Guide*. London: Palgrave Macmillan.

Gaffney-Rhys, R. & Jones, J. (2010). Issues surrounding the introduction of formal student contracts. *Assessment and Evaluation in Higher Education*. **35** (6), 711–25.

Galardl, K.M. (2012). *Importance of Support Services for On- and Off-Campus Graduate Students*. Online Submission (ERIC).

Gannon-Leary, P. & Smailes, J. (2009). Getting the most out of your conference experiences. *Red Guide No. 56*. University of Northumbria.

Gemmell, I., Sandars, J., Taylor, S. & Reed, K. (2011). Teaching science and technology via online distance learning: the experience of teaching biostatistics in an online Master of Public Health programme. *Open Learning*. **26** (2), 165–71.

Getman, J. & Reynolds, N. (2002). Ideas to action: ten hints for getting the most from a conference. *Educause Quarterly*. **3**, 58–60.

Gibbons, C. (2012). Stress, positive psychology and the National Student Survey. *Psychology Teaching Review*. **18** (2), 22–30.

Good, M. (2013). Publishing Your First Journal Article: an Academic Publisher's View – 1 http://blog.journals.cambridge.org/2013/05/publishing-your-first-journal-article-an-academic-publishers-view-1/ (Accessed 9 January 2014).

Grund, A., Brassler, N.K. & Fries, S. (2013). Torn between study and leisure: How motivational conflicts relate to students' academic and social adaptation. *Journal of Educational Psychology*. **106** (1), 242–57.

Hall, A. (2007). 'Turning your coursework into articles' in D.P.J. Soule, L. Whiteley & S. McIntosh (eds) *Writing for Scholarly Journals: Publishing in the Arts, Humanities and Social Sciences*. Glasgow: eSharp. 10–23.

Hartley, J. (2008). *Academic Writing and Publishing: A Practical Handbook*. Abingdon: Routledge.

Haslam, J. (2013a). How to get your book published, part 1. http://blog.journals.cambridge.org/2013/03/how-to-get-your-book-published-by-cambridge-university-press-part-1/ (Accessed 9 January 2014).

Haslam, J. (2013b). How to get your book published, part 2. http://blog.journals.cambridge.org/2013/03/how-to-get-your-book-published-part-2/ (Accessed 9 January 2014).

Haslam, J. (2013c). How to get your book published, part 3. http://blog.journals.cambridge.org/2013/03/how-to-get-your-book-published-part-3/ (Accessed 9 January 2014).

Higher Education Academy (HEA) (2013). *Using PRES to enhance the experience of postgraduate researchers: a good practice guide*. UK Higher Education Academy.

Hemingway, P. (2009). *What is a Systematic Review?* London: Hayward Medical Communications.

Herzberg, F. (1987). One more time: how do you motivate employees? Including a retrospective commentary (originally published in 1968). *Harvard Business Review*. **65** (5), 109–20.

Hesketh, A.J. & Knight, P.T. (1999). Postgraduates' choice of programme: helping universities to market and postgraduates to choose. *Studies in Higher Education*. **24** (2), 151–63.

Hill, H.S. & Hulya, J.Y. (2014). Bridging didactic, interdisciplinary service learning and practice in health professions education: students' perspectives. *Education+ Training*. **56** (5), 6.

Howell, G. & Buck, J. (2012). The adult student and course satisfaction: What matters most? *Innovative Higher Education*. **37** (3), 215–26.

Huberman, M. & Miles, M.B. (eds). (2002). *The Qualitative Researcher's Companion*. Thousand Oaks, CA: Sage.

Jacklin, A. & Le Riche, P. (2009). Reconceptualising student support: from 'support' to 'supportive'. *Studies in Higher Education*. **34** (7), 735–49.

Jancey, J. & Burns, S. (2013). Institutional factors and the postgraduate student experience. *Quality Assurance in Education*. **21** (3), 311–22.

Jefferies, A. & Skidmore, M. (2010). Evaluation of a collaborative mentorship program in a multi-site postgraduate training program. *Medical Teacher*. **32** (8), 695–97.

Jepsen, D.M. & Neumann, R. (2010). Undergraduate student intentions for postgraduate study. *Journal of Higher Education Policy and Management*. **32** (5), 455–66.

Kadivar, H. (2010). The importance of mentorship for success in family medicine. *The Annals of Family Medicine.* **8** (4), 374–75.

Kell, C. (2006). An analysis of entry-level postgraduate students' readiness for student-centred, Master's level learning. *Learning in Health and Social Care.* **5** (3), 133–41.

Kostovich, C., Saban, K. & Collins, E. (2010). Becoming a nurse researcher: Theimportance of mentorship. *Nursing Science Quarterly.* **23** (4), 281–86.

Larned, J.G. (2012). Becoming more resilient. *FBI Law Enforcement Bulletin.* **81** (10), 25–31.

Lave, J. & Wenger, E. (1991). *Situated Learning: Legitimate Peripheral Participation.* Cambridge: Cambridge University Press.

Marshall, M. & Gordon, F. (2010). Exploring the role of the interprofessional mentor. *Journal of Interprofessional Care.* **24** (4), 362–74.

Maslow, A.H. (1954). *Motivation and Personality.* New York: Harper.

Maslow, A.H. (1955). 'Deficiency motivation and growth motivation' in M.R. Jones (ed.) *Nebraska Symposium on Motivation.* Lincoln: University of Nebraska Press. 3, 1–30.

McDonald, K. (2011). Online Publishing and Plagiarism: Keeping Alert. http://www.vitae.ac.uk/researchers/346441-392041/Online-Publishing-and-Plagiarism-Keeping-Alert.html (Accessed 31 October 2013).

McClatchey, W. & Bridges, K.W. (2014). Lessons learned in development of an interdisciplinary science curriculum support organization. *Innovative Strategies for Teaching in the Plant Sciences.* New York: Springer. 21–31.

McMenamin, R., McGrath, M., Cantillon, P., & MacFarlane, A. (2014). Training socially responsive healthcare graduates: Is service learning an effective educational approach? *Medical Teacher.* **36** (4), 291–307.

Mizrachi, D. & Bates, M.J. (2013). Undergraduates' personal academic information management and the consideration of time and task-urgency. *Journal of the American Society for Information Science and Technology.* **64** (8), 1590–607.

Moriber, N.A., Wallace-Kazer, M., Shea, J., Grossman, S., Wheeler, K., & Conelius, J. (2014). Transforming doctoral education through the Clinical Electronic Portfolio. *Nurse Educator.* **39** (4), 153–205.

Mullins, G. & Kiley, M. (2002), 'It's a PhD, not a Nobel Prize': how experienced examiners assess research theses. *Studies in Higher Education.* **27** (4), 369–86.

Murphy, A. (2010). *Academic Writing and Publishing Matter for the Scholar-Researcher.* Dublin: Dublin Institute of Technology.

Murray, R. (2009). *Writing for Academic Journals.* 2nd edn. Berkshire: Open University Press.

Murray, R. & Moore, S. (2006). *The Handbook of Academic Writing: A Fresh Approach.* Maidenhead: Open University Press/McGraw-Hill.

Nash, S. & Scammell, J. (2009). How to use coaching and action learning to support mentors in the workplace. *Nursing Times.* **106** (3), 20–23.

National Union of Students. (2008). *NUS Student Experience Report.* London: NUS.

Neuman, L.W. (2002). *Social Research Methods: Qualitative and Quantitative Approaches.* Harlow, Essex: Pearson Educational.

Nikolova, I., Van Ruysseveldt, J., De Witte, H., & Syroit, J. (2014). Work-based learning: Development and valdation of a scale measuring the learning potential of the workplace (LPW). *Journal of Vocational Behavior.* **84** (1), 1–10.

Nursing and Midwifery Council (2010). *The NMC Code of Professional Conduct: Standards for Conduct, Performance and Ethics.* London: NMC.

Oxford English Dictionary (2014). http://www.oxforddictionaries.com/definition/english/empirical?q=empirical (Accessed 30 June 2014).

Park, Y.K., Song, J.H., Yoon, S.W., & Kim, J. (2014). Learning organization and innovative behavior: The mediating effect of work engagement. *European Journal of Training and Development.* **38** (1/2), 75–94.

Pearson, M. (2012). Building bridges: higher degree student retention and counselling support. *Journal of Higher Education Policy and Management.* **34** (2), 187–99.

Petticrew, M. & Roberts, H. (2003). Evidence, hierarchies, and typologies: horses for courses. *Journal of Epidemiological Community Health.* **57**, 527–29.

Pitman, T. (2000). Perceptions of academics and students as customers: A survey of administrative staff in higher education. *Journal of Higher Education Policy and Management.* **22** (2), 165–75.

Plowright, D. (2011) *Using Mixed Methods: Frameworks for an Integrated Methodology.* London: SAGE.

PRISMA (2009). Preferred Reporting Items for Systematic Reviews and Meta-Analyses. http://www.prisma-statement.org/index.htm (Accessed 30 June 2014).

Quality Assurance Agency for Higher Education (2008). *The Framework for Higher Education Qualifications in England, Wales and Northern Ireland.* UK: QAA.

Quality Assurance Agency for Higher Education (2010). *Master's Degree Characteristics, The Quality Assurance Agency for Higher Education.* QAA.

Research Excellence Framework (2014). http://www.ref.ac.uk/ (Accessed 18 November 2014).

Sandelowski, M., Docherty, S. & Emden, C. (1997). Focus on qualitative methods. Qualitative metasynthesis: issues and techniques. *Research in Nursing and Health.* **20**, 365–72.

Savio, N.D. & Nikolopoulos, K. (April–June 2013). A strategic forecasting framework for governmental decision-making and planning. *International Journal of Forecasting,* **29** (2), 311–21.

Smith, M. (2012). Publishing your work in an academic journal – three do's and a don't. http://blog.journals.cambridge.org/2012/11/publishing-your-work-in-an-academic-journal-three-dos-and-a-dont/ (Accessed 13 December 2013).

Smith, P. & Elliott, M. (1995). 'The Importance of Applied Research' in B. Smith & S. Brown (eds) *Research, Teaching and Learning in Higher Education.* SEDA (Society for Educational Development Association) & Kogan Page.

Snowden, D.J. & Boone, M.E. (2007). A leader's framework for decision-making, *Harvard Business Review.* **85** (11), 68–76.

Soles, D. (2010). *The Essentials of Academic Writing.* 2nd edn. Boston, USA: Wadsworth.

Sowan A.K. & Jenkins, L.S. (2013). Designing, delivering and evaluating a distance learning nursing course responsive to students' needs. *International Journal of Medical Informatics.* **82** (6), 553–64.

Thomas, A., Menon, A., Boruff, J., Rodriguez, A. M., & Ahmed, S. (2014). Applications of social constructivist learning theories in knowledge translation for healthcare professionals: a scoping review. *Implementation Science.* **9** (1), 54.

Thompson, J. & Bekhradnia, B. (2011). *Higher Education: Students at the Heart of the System: an Analysis of the Higher Education White Paper.* London: Higher Education Policy Institute.

Tobbell, J. & O'Donnell, V. (2013). Entering postgraduate study: A qualitative study of a neglected transition. *International Journal for Cross-Disciplinary Subjects in Education.* **4** (1).

UCLA (2014). Introduction to SAS. UCLA: Statistical Consulting Group. http://www.ats.ucla.edu/stat/sas/notes2/ (Accessed 30 June 2014).

UNISTATS, 2013-last update. http://unistats.direct.gov.uk/ (Accessed 10 January 2013).

Vankim, N.A. & Nelson, T.F. (2013). Vigorous physical activity, mental health, perceived stress, and socializing among college students. *American Journal of Health Promotion.* **28** (1), 7–15. https://www.vitae.ac.uk/ (Accessed 2 December 2014)

Vygotsky, L.S. (1978). *Mind in Society: The Development of High Psychological Processes.* Harvard University Press.

Wainwright, E. & Marandet, E. (2010). Parents in higher education: impacts of university learning on the self and the family. *Educational Review.* **62** (4), 449–65.

Wilkinson, D. (2005). *The Essential Guide to Postgraduate Study.* SAGE Study Skills, London: SAGE Publications.

Wisker, G. (2007). *The Postgraduate Research Handbook: Succeed with your MA, MPhil, EdD and PhD.* Basingstoke: Palgrave Macmillan.

Wisker, G., Robinson, G., Trafford, V., Warnes, M. & Creighton, E. (2003). From supervisory dialogues to successful PhDs: Strategies supporting and enabling the learning conversations of staff and students at postgraduate level. *Teaching in Higher Education.* **8** (3), 383–97.

Xiao, L., Wang, J. & Ferguson, M.K. (2014). Competence versus mastery: The time course for developing proficiency in video-assisted thoracoscopic lobectomy. *The Journal of Thoracic and Cardiovascular Surgery.* **147** (4), 1150–54.

Yadegaridehkordi, E., Iahad, N.A. & Ahmad, N. (2013). Collaborative learning tools in higher education: Literature review (2007–2012). *Australian Journal of Basic and Applied Sciences.* **7** (8), 285–96.

Useful resources

Higher Education Academy (HEA)

https://www.heacademy.ac.uk/

The Higher Education Academy champions excellent learning and teaching in higher education. It is an independent organisation, funded by the four UK higher education funding bodies and by subscriptions and grants. The HEA has published a number of best practice papers relating to postgraduate education.

Motivation

http://www.thersa.org

The Royal Society for the encouragement of Arts, Manufactures and Commerce (RSA) has produced a series of animations and you may find this one useful in the light of the discussion of motivation in Chapter 2.

RSA Animate – Drive: The surprising truth about what motivates us
http://www.youtube.com/results?search_query=the+surprising+truth+about+what+motivates+us&sm=1
(Accessed 9 March 2014).

National Postgraduate Committee (NPC)

http://www.npc.org.uk/

The NPC is a charity established to advance, in the public interest, postgraduate education in the UK. It is made up of postgraduate student representatives from various educational institutions. The NPC aims to promote the interests of postgraduates studying in the UK, holds an annual conference, and publishes guidelines and codes of practice.

PhD comics

http://phdcomics.com/comics.php

Piled Higher and Deeper (also known as PhD Comics) is a humorous newspaper and web comic strip, written and drawn by Jorge Cham, which follows the lives of several postgraduate students. First published in 1997, when Cham was a postgraduate student himself at Stanford University, the strip deals with issues of life for postgraduates, including the difficulties of scientific research, the perils of procrastination, the complex student–supervisor relationship and the endless search for free food.

The Postgraduate Forum

http://www.postgraduateforum.com/

The UK Postgraduate Forum is an online forum that has been set up to 'help current, future and previous postgraduate students to exchange ideas, get advice and generally help each other out.' You will find lots of discussion here about postgraduate studies.

Quality Assurance Agency (QAA)

http://www.qaa.ac.uk/

The Quality Assurance Agency for Higher Education aims to safeguard standards and improve the quality of UK higher education. The QAA offers 'advice, guidance and support to help UK universities, colleges and other institutions provide the best possible student experience of higher education'. The QAA also publishes a range of reference documents that promote best practice and standards.

Ranking journals

http://eigenfactor.org/

This useful website gives details of the impact of scholarly journals, and details of the key journals in most academic fields. It is interactive and provides a useful resource.

UK Council for Graduate Education (UKCGE)

https://www.ukcge.ac.uk/main/home

The UKCGE is an independent representative body for postgraduate education in the UK. Its mission is to be 'the authoritative voice for postgraduate education in the UK, providing high quality leadership and support to its members to promote a strong and sustainable postgraduate education sector.' The UKCGE produces best practice documents and runs regular events and conferences.

Useful websites

http://www.findamasters.com/
(Accessed 13 January 2013).

http://www.prospects.ac.uk/
(Accessed 7 January 2013).

http://www.jisc.ac.uk/media/documents/publications/reports/2010/managingexpectations.pdf
(Accessed 2 December 2014).

Vitae

http://www.vitae.ac.uk/

This useful website provides many valuable links for researchers, particularly to the various networks that can support and encourage your development as a researcher.

Index